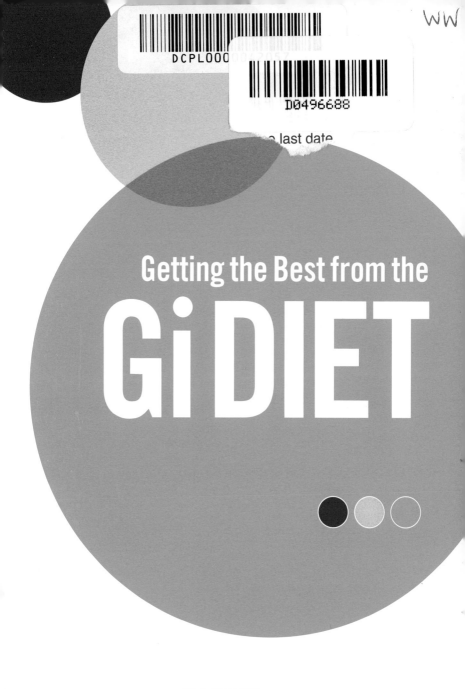

Getting the Best from the
Gi DIET

Virgin BOOKS

Rick Gallop

First published in Great Britain in 2008 by
Virgin Books Ltd
Thames Wharf Studios
Rainville Road
London
W6 9HA

Designed by Virgin Books Ltd

Printed and bound in Germany by APPL

Contents

INTRODUCTION   **4**

Part 1 – The Gi Diet: A Different Approach
1. Understanding weight loss – fats, proteins and carbohydrates   6
2. The Gi Diet – the basics   13
3. Losing weight on the Gi Diet   18

Part 2 – How to Follow the Gi Diet
4. Eating and shopping – the green-light way   26
5. Eating away from home   51
6. Cooking on the Gi Diet   57
7. Phase I – the 7-day plan   76
8. The green-light glossary   108

Part 3 – Your Future on the Gi Diet
9. Staying power – keeping yourself motivated   113
10. Exercise   117
11. Phase II   126
12. The Gi Diet and Health   129

Appendices   **138**

Index   **158**

Introduction

When my first book, *The Gi Diet*, was published back in 2002, I simply wanted to let people know about the fantastic method I'd found for losing weight – and keeping it off. Like many of you reading this book, I had tried all the diets going, but had never managed to shed those final pounds. I always failed to keep the weight off, because the diets left me feeling hungry and prone to temptation. When I developed my own Gi Diet, based on the simple traffic-light system for choosing which foods to eat, I was pleased that I could pass on this information to all those people in similar situations to me.

Little did I know that this book would be the first in a six-book series, which would go on to sell over 2 million copies in 22 countries. Of course I'm delighted, but my real pleasure is in knowing that my diet has really worked for so many people the world over.

The beauty of the Gi Diet is its simplicity. The way to permanent weight loss is here for you in black and white – or should I say red, yellow and green! Because the system for choosing food on the Gi Diet is as simple to follow as a set of traffic lights. There's no counting calories or points or any other complicated measurements involved. Just a few easy-to-remember principles, and a handily categorised list of all the foods you're likely to find on the supermarket shelves. It's so easy to follow that soon your new way of eating will become second nature – you won't even need to look at those shopping lists again! In fact, the Gi Diet is not so much a diet as a permanent change in the way you eat.

There are a lot of diets out there, but this is the only one that will guarantee you won't go hungry, get bored or give up because it's too complicated to follow. It really works, and the tens of thousands of emails I've received from happy readers is testament to that.

I've written books on all aspects of the Gi Diet, from the basic principles, to a pocket shopping and eating-out guide, a cookbook, a guide aimed at specifically women and families, and even an express version for busy people. But so far there's not one book that combines all these aspects into a single, easy-to-follow plan.

Until now. *Getting the Best from the Gi Diet* really does, in the words of that old cliché, exactly what it says on the tin. Here you'll find everything you need to know in order to follow the Gi Diet and lose weight healthily and permanently. But also a whole host of extras, from advice on cooking and preparing meals, to handy shopping lists, tips for eating away from home, preparing lunch boxes, not to mention some delicious recipes and a 7-day menu plan to get you started.

So what are you waiting for? Your future as a slimmer, more energetic, not to mention healthier you is waiting to be discovered between these pages. And I bet by the time you've mastered the basic principles, you won't even realise you're on a diet!

Enjoy.

1 Understanding Weight Loss – Fats, Proteins and Carbohydrates

WHY ARE WE BECOMING SO FAT?

It's impossible to open a paper or switch on the news nowadays without a story about Britain's 'obesity epidemic' jumping out at you. The statistics truly are astonishing: 60% of British adults today are overweight, but, even more worryingly, nearly one in five is defined as obese (seriously overweight); that's three times more than twenty years ago. How have we managed to put on so many pounds in such a short time?

While obesity is a complicated subject, affected by a whole variety of factors from the food we eat and our activity levels to genetics, there is nevertheless a simple reason for becoming overweight. We gain weight when we eat more calories than we burn. That is to say, consume too many calories and your body will store what it doesn't need in the form of fat.

So, where are our diets going wrong? In order to understand that, we need to look at the three main food groups – fats, proteins and carbohydrates – and how they are digested, absorbed and metabolised by our bodies.

FATS

For years, fat has been public enemy number one. Everyone from doctors and nutritionists to government officials has told us that the way to maintain a healthy weight is to eat a low-fat, high-carbohydrate diet.

So if you've ever tried to lose weight, you probably started by cutting down on fat. Instead of having a fry-up for breakfast, you switched to cornflakes with skimmed milk. Instead of eating a burger at lunch, you opted for chicken noodle soup and a slice of white bread without butter. Instead of grabbing a packet of crisps when you felt peckish, you snacked on rice cakes.

You may have felt virtuous about your healthy choices, but when weigh-day came, and you eagerly stepped on the scales ... you'd gained another two pounds! What went wrong?

The surprising truth is, fat consumption in this country has remained virtually constant over the past ten years, yet obesity numbers have rocketed. Obviously, fat isn't totally to blame.

That said, I'm not giving you a free rein to eat all the fatty foods you want. Most fats can be quite harmful to your health. It's alarming to read some of the popular diet books on the market today and find that they advocate eating lots of cream, cheese and steak. These foods are all high in saturated fat (see below), which can thicken and harden your arteries, leading to heart attack and stroke. There is also increasing evidence that colon and prostate cancer as well as Alzheimer's are associated with high levels of saturated fats.

While eating a low-fat diet is good, no-fat is not an option. Fats are essential for the digestive process, cell development and overall health. Despite their bad reputation, certain fats are essential to your overall diet, health and well-being.

However, if you're concerned about your weight, be aware that the quantity of fat you consume makes a huge difference. Fat has more than twice the calories per gram than either carbohydrates or proteins.

There are different types of fat, which I have grouped under the headings 'bad fats', 'really ugly fats', 'acceptable fats' and 'best fats'.

Bad fats

Saturated fats are certainly 'bad' fats. You can recognise them because they're solid at room temperature and almost always come from animal sources. The two exceptions to this rule are coconut oil and palm oil – these two vegetable oils are also saturated. Because these oils are cheap, you'll find them in many snack foods, especially biscuits.

Really ugly fats

Hydrogenated oils are vegetable oils that have been heat-treated to make them harder and thicker. Hydrogenated oils (and also partially hydrogenated oils) are our main source of trans fats, and are potentially the most dangerous to our health. Trans fats (or trans fatty acids) have all the worst characteristics of saturated fats, and possibly more. So don't use spreads containing them and avoid foods whose labels list hydrogenated or partially hydrogenated oils among their ingredients. Many biscuits, crackers, cereals, baked goods and fast foods contain these really ugly fats.

Fortunately, many manufacturers are removing hydrogenated, partially hydrogenated and trans fats from their products, and several of the big supermarkets are doing the same with their own brand lines.

Acceptable fats

'Acceptable' fats are the polyunsaturated fats, which are cholesterol free. Most of the familiar vegetable oils, such as corn and sunflower, fall into this category.

Another kind of highly beneficial oil, which is a polyunsaturated fat, but in a category of its own, is a group called omega-3 fatty acids. Theses oils can help lower cholesterol and protect your cardiovascular health. They are found in oily fish such as salmon, trout, mackerel, tuna and herring, as well as in walnuts, flaxseed and rapeseed oils. Some brands of eggs also contain omega-3 oils.

The best fats

The 'best' fats are monounsaturated fats, which are found in foods like olives, peanuts, almonds and olive and rapeseed oils. Monounsaturated fats actually have a beneficial effect on cholesterol and are good for your heart, so try to incorporate them into your diet and look for them on food labels.

Interestingly, monounsaturates are one reason why the incidence of heart disease is low in Mediterranean countries, where olive oil is a staple. Although fancy olive oil is expensive, you can enjoy the same health benefits from less costly supermarket brands. It doesn't have to be extra-virgin, cold-pressed.

PROTEINS

Over the years, a lot of nonsense and misinformation has been written about protein and its role in our diet. For a long time, nutritionists and dieticians didn't think protein was a factor in weight control. Then, in the 1970s, high-protein diets suddenly became fashionable. You could supposedly eat all the protein and fat you liked, while minimising your carbohydrate intake.

This type of low-carb diet has become all the rage once again, but as we know by now, it's harmful to your health and does nothing to reduce fat cells. High-protein diets have rightly been criticised by nutritionists and doctors alike.

Most people would agree (and rightly so) that protein is important. It's an essential part of your diet. In fact, you are already half composed of proteins: 50% of your dry body weight is made up of muscles, organs, skin and hair, and all of these are made from these vital building blocks.
Proteins are required for growth (building body tissues) and repairing (body maintenance). They also play a role in nearly all metabolic reactions.

Our brains need proteins, too. Proteins are used to synthesise neurotransmitters – chemicals that transmit messages in the brain and around the nervous system.

Protein is also much more effective than carbohydrates or fat in satisfying hunger – a meal or snack containing protein leaves you feeling satisfied and nicely full. This means it also helps you to lose weight or maintain a healthy weight. Because it takes time for your body to digest, absorb and metabolise protein, you feel fuller, for longer – and this 'fuller, longer' principle is key to the Gi Diet's success.

The type of protein you consume is important, though. Proteins are found in a broad range of food products, both animal and vegetable, and not just in the familiar sources like red meat and whole dairy products, which are high in saturated or 'bad' fat.

Sources of protein
Most of the protein in our diet comes from animal sources: meat (including poultry), fish and other seafood, dairy products such as milk, yoghurt and cheese, and eggs.

We can also get protein from vegetable sources such as pulses (beans and lentils) and soya-based products such as tofu.

Animal protein is easy for the body to utilise, but it has a downside, too. Many forms of animal protein (especially red meat, and full-fat dairy products) are high in saturated fats (see page 7), which are harmful to your health, especially your heart. This is why the medical field is so concerned about the continued popularity of high-protein/low-carb diets like Atkins. High protein per se is not so much of a problem as the fact that most people following these diets tend to get most of their protein from high-fat animal proteins such as red meat, sending their saturated fat intake sky high – with all the health concerns this brings.

So what sort of protein should you be including in your diet?

Animal sources:
• Lean or low-fat cuts of meat that have been trimmed of any visible fat
• Skinless poultry
• Fresh, frozen or canned fish (but not the kind that's coated with batter, which is invariably high in fat)
• Low-fat milk products such as skimmed milk
• Low-fat fruit yoghurt with sweetener, such as Splenda®
• Low-fat cottage cheese
• Egg whites

Vegetable sources:
• Pulses (beans and lentils)
• Tofu
• Nuts and seeds
• Soya powder or unflavoured whey protein powder, which is great for sprinkling in or on meals if they're otherwise lacking in protein

Nutritionally speaking, pulses (beans and lentils) are hard to beat – they're just about a perfect food. Pulses are high in protein and fibre, and low in saturated fat.

We need to wise up to the wonders of beans and lentils. In the UK, they're rather overlooked, in favour of animal protein, but if we look around the world's cuisines, we see a huge array of tasty ways to cook them – we've no excuse!

Nuts and seeds are two more excellent sources of protein. They're relatively low in fat, and the fat they do contain is mainly the heart-healthy unsaturated kind. However, they're not a low-fat food, and the calories can add up if you eat a whole bowlful, particularly as they're so moreish!

One of the most important things about protein is to spread your daily allowance across all your meals. Too often we grab a hasty breakfast of coffee and toast – a protein-free meal. Lunch is sometimes not much of an improvement: a bowl of pasta with vegetables or a green salad with French bread. Where's your protein? A typical afternoon snack of a cake or biscuit, perhaps with a piece of fruit, contains not a gram of protein. Generally, it's not until dinner that we include protein in our meal, usually our entire daily recommended allowance – and some.

Remember that protein is a critical brain food, providing amino acids for the neurotransmitters that relay messages in the brain. This means it's better to load up on protein earlier in the day rather than later. That way your mind will be more alert and active for your daily activities.

However, as I have said, the best solution is to spread your protein consumption throughout the day. This will help keep you on the ball and feeling full.

Quick protein checklist:
• Space your protein intake throughout the day. Include some protein in all your meals and snacks.
• Eat only low-fat protein, preferably from both animal and vegetable sources.

CARBOHYDRATES

As I've already mentioned, our fat and protein consumption has not changed significantly over the past decade, yet the percentage of overweight people in the population has soared. What's changed? Well, the answer lies in something you've probably never thought of as fattening at all – and that's grain. Have you noticed the ever-increasing number of supermarket shelves devoted to products made from flour, corn and rice? Our stores now have huge biscuit and snack-food sections; whole aisles of breakfast cereals; numerous shelves of pastas and noodles; and baskets and baskets of bagels, rolls, muffins and loaves of bread.

Since grain is a carbohydrate, let's look at this third component of our diet, and whether carbs deserve their bad rap.

Our ever-increasing demand for these kinds of carbs helps explain why over half of British adults are overweight, and why 1 in 5 are considered obese – triple the number 20 years ago!

Eating too much grain is certainly half of the problem. The rest is the type of grain we're eating, which is generally highly processed. Flour is a good example. While, traditionally, grain was ground between grinding stones, modern high-speed flour mills use steel rollers to produce an extraordinarily finely ground product. The whole wheat is steamed and scarified by tiny razor-sharp blades to remove the bran (the source of most of the fibre in the grain) and the endosperm. Then the wheat germ (where most of the protein is found) and oil are removed because they turn rancid too quickly and reduce the product's shelf life. What's left after all that processing is then bleached and marketed as white flour. This is what almost all the breads, rolls, bagels, muffins, biscuits, cereals and pastas we consume are made of. Even many 'brown' breads are simply artificially coloured white bread!

And it's not just flour that's highly processed nowadays. A hundred years ago, most of the food people ate came straight from the farm to the fork. Before everyone had refrigerators, and with little knowledge of food chemistry, most food remained unprocessed and in its original state. However, advances in science, along with the migration of many women out of the kitchen and into the workforce, led to a revolution in prepared foods.

Now everything is tailored to make things quick and easy for us. We have instant rice, noodles and potatoes, as well as entire meals that are ready to eat after just a few minutes in the microwave.

What's the problem? Well ... the more a food is processed beyond its natural state, the less processing your body has to do to digest it. And the quicker you digest your food, the sooner you are hungry again and the more you tend to eat. Think of the difference between eating a bowl of old-fashioned porridge oats and a bowl of sugary breakfast cereal. The oatmeal stays with you – it 'sticks to your ribs' as my mother used to say – whereas you are reaching for a croissant only an hour after eating the bowl of sugary cereal.

Our fundamental problem, then, is that we are eating foods that are far too easy for our bodies to digest – with these processed foods, a lot of the work is already done before they even reach our digestive systems.

We obviously can't turn back the clock to simpler times, but we need to somehow slow down the digestive process so we don't feel hungry again so soon. The solution? We have to eat foods that are slow-release, and that break down at a slow and steady rate in our digestive system, leaving us feeling fuller for longer.

This is the basis for the Gi Diet, which I'll explain in more detail in the following chapter.

2 The Gi Diet – the Basics

FINDING THE SLOW-RELEASE FUELS

As mentioned at the end of the previous chapter, the key to losing weight is to eat 'slow-release' foods that are broken down steadily and keep you filled up for longer.

The principal tool in identifying these slow-release foods is the glycemic index, or Gi, which is the basis of the Gi Diet.

THE GLYCEMIC INDEX (GI)

The glycemic index measures the speed at which foods are digested and converted into glucose, which is the body's source of energy. The faster a food breaks down, the higher its rating on the glycemic index, which sets sugar at 100 and scores all other foods against that number.

Here are just a few examples:

Food	GI	Food	GI
Sugar	100	Popcorn (plain)	55
Baguette	95	Orange	44
Rice	87	All Bran	43
Cornflakes	84	Porridge	42
Potatoes (baked)	84	Spaghetti	41
Doughnut	76	Tomato	38
Cheerios	75	Apple	38
Bagel	72	Yoghurt (low-fat)	33
Raisins	64	Fettuccine	32
Rice (basmati)	58	Beans	31
Muffin (bran)	56	Grapefruit	25
Potatoes (new, boiled)	56	Yoghurt (fat-free with sweetener)	14

The Glycemic Index has exciting implications for anyone who wishes to lose weight. It has been proven that keeping glucose levels low is the key to permanent weight loss. It's also an extremely useful tool for anyone wanting to eat healthily.

This is how it works: when you eat a high-Gi food, such as white bread, your body rapidly converts it into glucose. The glucose dissolves in your bloodstream and spikes its glucose level, giving you that 'sugar high'. The chart below illustrates the impact of digesting sugar on the level of glucose in your bloodstream compared to split peas, which have a low Gi rating.

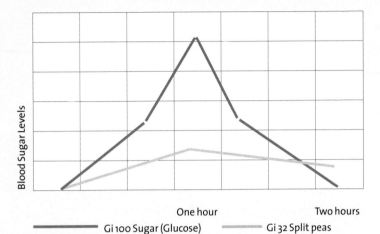

Blood Sugar Levels

One hour   Two hours

Gi 100 Sugar (Glucose)   Gi 32 Split peas

As you can see, there is a dramatic difference between the two. What is also apparent from the chart is that after your glucose level spikes, the sugar quickly disappears from your bloodstream, leaving you feeling starved of energy and looking for more fuel. Something most of us experience regularly is the feeling of lethargy that follows an hour or so after a fast-food lunch, which generally consists of high-Gi foods. The surge of glucose followed by the rapid drain leaves us feeling sluggish, lethargic and hungry. So what do we do? Around mid-afternoon, we look for a quick sugar fix, or snack, to bring us out of the slump. A few biscuits or a bag of crisps – also high-Gi foods – cause another rush of glucose, which again disappears a short time later. Leaving you convinced you need another biscuit, as the vicious yo yo cycle continues.

Eating a diet of high-Gi foods will make you feel hungry more often and you will end up eating more as a result – and probably gaining weight.

Low-Gi foods, on the other hand, are the tortoise to the high-Gi foods' hare. Your digestive system breaks them down at a slow, steady rate. Tortoise-like, they stay the course, sustaining you and making you feel full longer. As a result, in the long run, you consume less food and fewer calories, without going hungry or feeling unsatisfied.

Slow-release, low-Gi carbohydrates help curb your appetite by leaving you feeling fuller for longer. When you combine them with lean protein and the best fats, which also help slow the digestive process, you have the magic combination that will allow you to maintain a healthy weight, or lose it if you need to, without feeling deprived.

UNDERSTANDING BLOOD SUGAR

The key player in the blood-sugar balance is insulin, a hormone secreted by the pancreas. Insulin does two things very well. First, it regulates the amount of sugar (glucose) in our bloodstream, removing the excess and diverting it into various body tissues for immediate short-term use, storing it as glycogen for immediate use by our muscles, or putting it into long-term storage as fat.

Second, it inhibits the conversion of body fat back into glucose for the body to burn. It acts as a security guard at the fat gates, only giving up its reserves reluctantly. So fat is easy to acquire and hard to lose. (Or, as they say, a second on the lips, for ever on the hips.) This evolutionary feature is a throwback to the days when our ancestors were hunter-gatherers, habitually experiencing times of feast or famine. When food was in abundance, the body stored its surplus as fat to tide it over the days when there wouldn't be much to eat. Insulin was the champion in this process, both helping to accumulate fat and then guarding its depletion when times were hard and food was short.

Eating high-Gi foods stimulates our bodies to release insulin, because, if our blood-sugar levels were allowed to rise unchecked, we would develop dangerous hyperglycaemia (high blood sugar). Insulin's job is to reduce the sugar levels in our blood and return them to the proper levels. If we don't need all that energy straight away, the glucose is squirrelled away as fat.

And soon we become hungry again. Our body will either draw on our reserves of fat and laboriously convert them back to sugar, or it will look for more food. Giving up extra fat is the body's last choice – who knows when that supply might come in handy! So your body would rather send you to the fridge for a new blood-sugar boost, than work to convert fat back to sugar. This helped our ancestors to survive back in the old days, but now it can lead to us piling on the pounds.

What we should do is limit the amount of insulin circulating in our system by avoiding high-Gi foods and instead choosing low-Gi foods. This will keep the supply of sugar in our bloodstream steady and consistent.

So, aside from the fact that they don't satisfy your hunger, there is a second reason why you should avoid eating high-Gi foods – they cause a spike of insulin, which, as well as promoting fat gain, can also contribute to other health problems.

THE TRAFFIC-LIGHT SYSTEM

Now that you have a little grounding in the science of the Gi Diet, let's get down to the nitty-gritty: what to eat and what to avoid.

How can you make the Gi Diet 'real'? Translated into actual food, what will you be eating? Well, for dinner you could have a grilled chicken breast (without the skin, which is full of fat), boiled new potatoes, a side salad of cos lettuce and red pepper, dressed with a little olive oil and lemon, and some asparagus if you feel like it. The trick is to stick to foods that have a low Gi, are low in fat (particularly saturated fat) and less calorie dense. This sounds – and, in fact, is – quite complex. And it also sounds as if I'm breaking my promise of simplicity. But don't worry: I've done all the calculations, measurements and maths for you, and sorted the foods you like to eat into easy-to-follow, traffic-light colours.

Here's how the colour-coded categories work:

Red-light foods: Avoid these. They are the high-Gi, higher-calorie foods.

Yellow-light foods: The foods in the yellow column are mid-range-Gi foods and should only be eaten when you've reached your target weight.

Green-light foods: This column lists foods that are low Gi, low in fat and lower in calories. These are the foods that will help you lose weight if you need to. But don't expect them to be tasteless and boring!

(To find out what to eat and what to avoid, check out the Complete Gi Diet Food Guide on pages 138–50.)

There are two phases in the Gi Diet: Phase I is for if you need to lose weight, and, during this time, you should stick to green-light foods, and avoid red-light and yellow-light foods. Once you've reached your target weight, and you wish to maintain it, you enter Phase II, or the way you will eat for the rest of your life. In Phase II, you can begin to enjoy yellow-light foods from time to time. I'll explain more about Phases I and II later in this book.

If you're a veteran of the low-carbohydrate craze, you'll be surprised to find potatoes and rice in the green-light column, but they are fine as long as they are the right type. Baked potatoes and French fries have a high-Gi value, while boiled, small new potatoes have a low-Gi value. Rice comes in different types, too. The short-grain, glutinous variety served in Chinese and Thai restaurants is high Gi, while long-grain, brown, basmati and wild rice are low Gi. Pasta is also a green-light food – as long as it is cooked only until al dente (with some firmness to the bite, rather than soft or soggy).

Any processing of food, including cooking, will increase its Gi rating, since heat breaks down a food's starch capsules and fibre, giving your digestive juices a head start, and hastening that rise in your blood sugar. This is why you should never overcook pasta or rice. The same holds true for vegetables; you should steam them or boil/microwave them in a small amount of water until they are just tender. This way, they will retain their vitamins and other nutrients, and their Gi rating will remain low.

Try to eat regularly throughout the day, with three main meals and three snacks. If you skimp on breakfast and lunch, you will probably be starving by dinner and pile on the food then. Have one snack mid-morning, another mid-afternoon and one before bed. The idea is to keep your digestive system happily busy so you won't start craving those red-light snacks.

Now that you know how the Gi Diet works, it's time to get started. In the next chapter, we've outlined the steps for beginning Phase I.

Summary:
1. The key to losing weight is to eat low-Gi, low-calorie foods.
2. Low-Gi foods are slower to digest, so you feel satisfied longer.
3. In Phase I, eat only green-light foods.
4. Eat three balanced meals and three snacks per day.

3 Losing Weight on the Gi Diet

WHY DO YOU WANT TO LOSE WEIGHT?

Whether you want to lose 10 pounds or 100, the Gi Diet can help. Perhaps you just want to drop a dress size or two, or your doctor has advised you to shed some pounds. It's important to look at the reasons why you or members of your family want to lose weight, as your answer will have a lot to do with your motivation to start and, more importantly, to stay the course.

Let's look at the most common reasons why people want to lose weight and see how they reflect your own.

1. Wanting to look better

Judging from the correspondence I have received – 25,000 emails and counting – the day when people discover that they can fit into their 'skinny' jeans again is at least as rewarding as seeing the reading on the bathroom scales falling. Most of us would rather shop for clothes that flatter and show off our bodies than resort to camouflage.

It's a powerful motivator when you walk into a room and a friend says, 'Have you lost weight? You look terrific!'

Weight loss boosts self-esteem and confidence, for women in particular, which in turn makes it easier to maintain new eating habits. It's amazing the difference the loss of just a few pounds can make, not only to how you look in your clothes but to how you feel about yourself.

And the evidence of the Gi Diet speaks for itself. I've sold more books based on word of mouth – people asking Gi Diet readers how they lost their weight – than through any other marketing strategy.

But remember that losing weight is not about trying to live up to unreachable, red-carpet standards of beauty or size-zero thinness; it's about feeling at ease in your body and liking what you see in the mirror.

2. Wanting more energy, and to feel less lethargic

Perhaps the most frequent comment I get from readers, apart from the thrill of losing pounds or going down a dress size, is the buzz of energy that comes with their new lighter, healthier body.

A while ago, I witnessed a dramatic demonstration of how much of an energy-sapper extra weight can be. My wife and I had just completed some house renovations to suit our empty-nest lifestyle, and as we were restoring some order, I asked Ruth to carry a couple of 20-pound dumb-bells up a flight of stairs to my new workout room. She could only get them to the first-floor landing before she had to put them down again. 'How do people who are 40 pounds overweight get around, let alone climb stairs?' she wondered. And 40 pounds of extra weight is not something you can just put down like a pair of dumb-bells when you want to. Imagine the energy that goes into carrying those pounds all the time!

That's the energy that will be available to you again if you shed any excess weight you're carrying.

Readers also tell me how thrilled they are when they find themselves able to do more exercise and to enjoy activities they might not have participated in since their teens. If regaining your former energy and vitality is important to you, you'll receive constant motivation as your new, lighter body rejoices in its recently acquired freedom to run, swim, play squash, or engage in any activity you may have given up for 'lack of energy'.

3. Wanting to be healthier, and to help your family become healthier

Even if health may not be your primary reason for losing weight, it is ultimately the most vital one. Being overweight and eating a poor diet are by far the most critical factors in increasing your chances of developing major diseases that can either undermine your quality of life or drastically shorten it. These serious conditions include heart disease, stroke, cancer, diabetes and Alzheimer's. Of course, your genes play an important role in your risk of these diseases, too, but anyone who is overweight and under-nourished must realise that they're greatly increasing their risk for these conditions.

The prospect of a long life, especially one free of pain, disability and disease, is a powerful motivator.

Keeping in mind these three incentives – looking and feeling better, enjoying greater energy and improving your overall health – will go a long way in helping you stick to the Gi Diet. I'll go as far as to say it will open up a whole new chapter in your life.

HOW MUCH SHOULD I WEIGH?

In this age of excessively and often unhealthily skinny supermodels and TV stars, it's easy to lose sight of what is a healthy weight. Every part of you, your skin, bones, organs, hair – everything – contributes to your total weight. But the only part that you want to reduce is your excess fat, so it's fatness, not weight, that is what we have to determine.

There have been many techniques designed to measure excess fatness, from measuring pinches of fat (which can be quite misleading) to convoluted formulas and tables requiring complex maths. Since everyone has a distinct body type, metabolism and genes, there are no absolute rules for how much you should weigh. The only accepted international standard for weight is the Body Mass Index (BMI), which is basically a measurement of how much you weigh relative to your height, and provides a pretty accurate estimate of whether you're a healthy weight or not.

On pages 22–23 is a BMI table that is very simple to use.

To find your BMI:
Find your height in the horizontal column at the top.
Find your weight in the vertical column on the left side.
Your BMI is where the two columns intersect.

BMI 19–24 = healthy weight range
BMI 25–29 = overweight
BMI 30+ = obese

Let's look at a couple of examples:

Sara is 5'6" and weighs 11st 7lb (73kg). That makes her BMI 26, which is four notches above her target BMI of 22. So, Sara needs to lose 1st 11lb (11.35kg) in order to bring her to her 22 BMI goal of 9st 10lb (62kg).

Will is 6'0" and weighs 13st 10lb (87kg). His BMI is also 26, but he needs to lose 1 stone (6.35kg) to bring his BMI down to his target level of 24 of 12st 10lbs (81kg).

The 1st 11lb that Sara has to shed and the 1 stone that Will needs to lose are pounds of fat – Sara's and Will's energy storage tanks. In order for them to lose weight, they must access and draw down those fat cells.

Too thin or too heavy is not good. Your health is at risk if your BMI falls below 18.5 or above 25. Women, who generally have a lower muscle mass and smaller frame than men, might want to aim towards the lower end of the healthy weight range, while men should generally aim at the higher end. However, if you are under 18, elderly or heavily muscled, these ratings do not apply to you (Governor Schwarzenegger wouldn't fit on the chart, and neither would tennis star Serena Williams. Professional rugby players would be classed as obese!). If you are over 65, then allow yourself 4.5kg (10lb) extra as that reserve may be helpful in cushioning a fall or if you become ill for a lengthy period when it may be difficult to eat.

As I said before, there are no absolute rules for how much you should weigh. Use this only as a guide, not as an absolute number. Nevertheless, it's a good general measure and the only one that has been accepted as an international standard. But, ultimately, it is up to you to decide what weight is right for you.

Your waist measurement

The other measurement you should concern yourself with is your waist measurement. This is an even better predictor of your health than your weight is. Abdominal fat is more than just an added weight problem. Recent research has shown that abdominal fat acts almost like a separate organ in the body, except this 'organ' is destructive, in that it releases harmful proteins and free fatty acids into the rest of the body, which can increase your risk of heart disease, stroke, cancer and diabetes. People who are 'apple-shaped' and store their fat around their waists are more likely to suffer health problems due to their abdominal fat than 'pear shapes' who put on weight around their hips, bottoms and thighs.

You are at risk of endangering your health if your waist measurement exceeds a certain size:

Increased risk for females: 35" (87.5cm) or more
Increased risk for males: 37" (92.5cm) or more

Seriously increased risk for females: 37" (92.5cm) or more
Seriously increased risk for males: 40" (100cm) or more

To measure your waist, put a tape measure around your waist at its widest, usually just above the navel level until it fits snugly, but isn't cutting into your flesh. Do not adopt the walk-down-the-beach-suck-in-your-tummy routine. Just stand naturally. There's no point in trying to fudge the numbers because the only person you're kidding is yourself.

An equally important measurement is your waist to hip measurement. For women this should be 0.85 or less and for men 0.95 or less. To find your ratio, simply divide your hip into your waist measurement. For example, a measurement of 44" hips and 36" waist would give an acceptable ration of 0.82.

BMI TABLE

WEIGHT				HEIGHT																		
BRITISH		US		FT INS																		
STONES	LBS	POUNDS	KILOS CM	4'6" 137	4'8" 142	4'10" 147	5'0" 152	5'2" 157	5'3" 160	5'4" 163	5'5" 165	5'6" 168	5'7" 170	5'8" 173	5'9" 175	5'10" 178	5'11" 180	6'0" 183	6'2" 188	6'4" 193	6'6" 198	6'8" 203
6	7	91	41	22.0	20.4	19.0	17.8	16.6	16.1	15.6	15.1	14.7	14.3	13.8	13.4	13.1	12.7	12.3	11.7	11.1	10.5	10.0
6	10	94	43	22.7	21.1	19.6	18.4	17.2	16.7	16.1	15.6	15.2	14.7	14.3	13.9	13.5	13.1	12.7	12.1	11.4	10.9	10.3
7	0	98	44	23.7	22.0	20.5	19.1	17.9	17.4	16.8	16.3	15.8	15.3	14.9	14.5	14.1	13.7	13.3	12.6	11.9	11.3	10.8
7	3	101	46	24.4	22.6	21.1	19.7	18.5	17.9	17.3	16.8	16.3	15.8	15.4	14.9	14.5	14.1	13.7	13.0	12.3	11.7	11.1
7	7	105	48	25.4	23.5	21.9	20.5	19.2	18.6	18.0	17.5	16.9	16.4	16.0	15.5	15.1	14.6	14.2	13.5	12.8	12.1	11.5
7	10	108	49	26.1	24.2	22.6	21.1	19.8	19.1	18.5	18.0	17.4	16.9	16.4	15.9	15.5	15.1	14.6	13.9	13.1	12.5	11.9
8	0	112	51	27.1	25.1	23.4	21.9	20.5	19.8	19.2	18.6	18.1	17.5	17.0	16.5	16.1	15.6	15.2	14.4	13.6	12.9	12.3
8	3	115	52	27.8	25.8	24.0	22.5	21.0	20.4	19.7	19.1	18.6	18.0	17.5	17.0	16.5	16.0	15.6	14.8	14.0	13.3	12.6
8	7	119	54	28.8	26.7	24.9	23.2	21.8	21.1	20.4	19.8	19.2	18.6	18.1	17.6	17.1	16.6	16.1	15.3	14.5	13.8	13.1
8	10	122	55	29.5	27.4	25.5	23.8	22.3	21.6	20.9	20.3	19.7	19.1	18.5	18.0	17.5	17.0	16.5	15.7	14.9	14.1	13.4
9	3	129	59	31.1	28.9	27.0	25.2	23.6	22.9	22.1	21.5	20.8	20.2	19.6	19.0	18.5	18.0	17.5	16.6	15.7	14.9	14.2
9	7	133	60	32.1	29.8	27.8	26.0	24.3	23.6	22.8	22.1	21.5	20.8	20.2	19.6	19.1	18.5	18.0	17.1	16.2	15.4	14.6
9	10	136	62	32.9	30.5	28.4	26.6	24.9	24.1	23.3	22.6	22.0	21.3	20.7	20.1	19.5	19.0	18.4	17.5	16.6	15.7	14.9
10	0	140	64	33.8	31.4	29.3	27.3	25.6	24.8	24.0	23.3	22.6	21.9	21.3	20.7	20.1	19.5	19.0	18.0	17.0	16.2	15.4
10	3	143	65	34.6	32.1	29.9	27.9	26.2	25.3	24.5	23.8	23.1	22.4	21.7	21.1	20.5	19.9	19.4	18.4	17.4	16.5	15.7
10	7	147	67	35.5	33.0	30.7	28.7	26.9	26.0	25.2	24.5	23.7	23.0	22.4	21.7	21.1	20.5	19.9	18.9	17.9	17.0	16.1
10	10	150	68	36.3	33.6	31.3	29.3	27.4	26.6	25.7	25.0	24.2	23.5	22.8	22.2	21.5	20.9	20.3	19.3	18.3	17.3	16.5
11	0	154	70	37.2	34.5	32.2	30.1	28.2	27.3	26.4	25.6	24.9	24.1	23.4	22.7	22.1	21.5	20.9	19.8	18.7	17.8	16.9
11	3	157	71	37.9	35.2	32.8	30.7	28.7	27.8	26.9	26.1	25.3	24.6	23.9	23.2	22.5	21.9	21.3	20.2	19.1	18.1	17.2
11	7	161	73	38.9	36.1	33.6	31.4	29.4	28.5	27.6	26.8	26.0	25.2	24.5	23.8	23.1	22.5	21.8	20.7	19.6	18.6	17.7
11	10	164	74	39.6	36.8	34.3	32.0	29.9	29.1	28.2	27.3	26.5	25.7	24.9	24.2	23.5	22.9	22.2	21.1	20.0	19.0	18.0
12	0	168	76	40.6	37.7	35.1	32.8	30.7	29.8	28.8	28.0	27.1	26.3	25.5	24.8	24.1	23.4	22.8	21.6	20.4	19.4	18.5
12	3	171	78	41.3	38.3	35.7	33.4	31.3	30.3	29.4	28.5	27.6	26.8	26.0	25.3	24.5	23.8	23.2	22.0	20.8	19.8	18.8
12	7	175	79	42.3	39.2	36.6	34.2	32.0	31.0	30.0	29.1	28.2	27.4	26.6	25.8	25.1	24.4	23.7	22.5	21.3	20.2	19.2

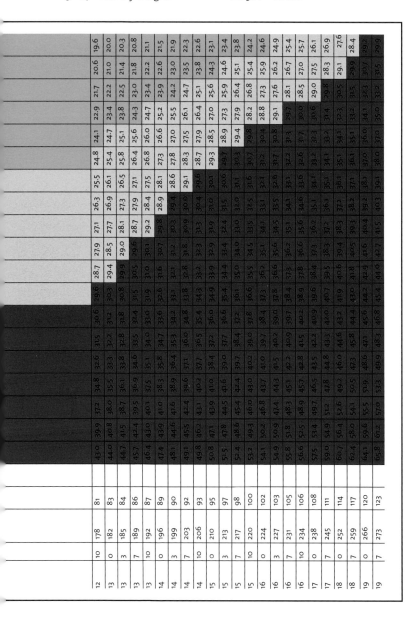

Setting your target

Once you know your BMI and waist measurement, and have set you're BMI and weight targets, you can get started.

If you want to lose weight, you need to begin with Phase I of the Gi Diet. If your BMI and waist measurement are fine, and you just want to keep them that way and maintain the health benefits of the Gi way of eating, then you can relax a little with Phase II. You'll learn more about Phase II in Chapter 11, but don't go there yet – bear with me while I just explain the basics. I promise it'll be worth it!

To help you chart your progress and keep track of the measurements you lose, you'll find a Weight and Waist Log for you to photocopy (Appendix VI). This can be a powerful motivator, since nothing is more encouraging than success.

But don't get obsessed with numbers on the scale – inches matter more, since they measure that crucial belly fat. Many people find themselves losing inches before they register any weight loss on the scales. Clothes start feeling a little looser, and, before you know it, you are down a dress size or slipping into your old jeans. Soon you will probably have to buy new clothes. My readers often tell me that I should have warned them about the extra cost of refurbishing their wardrobe!

WHY OTHER DIETS DON'T WORK

If losing weight has so many obvious benefits, why the obesity crisis? Why is the prevalence of overweight and obesity climbing year on year, especially as there are hundreds of new diet books flooding into the bookshops all the time? The simple fact is that most diets don't work. And the reason they fail is that people don't stick to them. Why do they give up? I'm sure the following explanations will be familiar to you.

Hunger

Many diets leave you feeling hungry, weak and deprived. Your stomach growls as you stagger through the day, and sooner or later you cave in and order a pizza with double cheese.

This feeling of perpetual hunger is the number-one reason for people's diets failing.

Inconvenience

The diet is too complicated and time-consuming to follow. You spend each day weighing and measuring food, calculating carbs or calories and keeping food diaries. Perhaps this is fun initially, but then it all just becomes a burden. Life is too busy to follow a diet that feels more like a maths exam.

Malnutrition

Many diets cut out essential nutrients, leaving you feeling lethargic, lacking energy and concerned about your health. Is it little wonder people give up if dieting makes them feel worse, not better?

The Gi Diet meets each of these barriers head on.

> • Low Gi green light foods ensure you won't go hungry or feel deprived
> • The traffic-light colour coding means you'll never have to count another calorie or point again
> • The inclusion of foods from all the principal food groups ensures a healthy and nutritious diet

It's not so much a diet as a new way of eating for the rest of your life. Losing weight and keeping it off has never been so easy.

4 Eating and Shopping – the Green-Light Way

To recap, if you're trying to lose weight, you'll need to follow Phase I of the Gi Diet, eating only green-light foods. Once you're at your target weight, or if you're already there, you can move on to Phase II (see Chapter 11), introducing yellow-light foods and slightly larger portions.

But before you dive in, there are many principles and hints that apply to the Gi Diet, whatever Phase you are on. Don't be tempted to skip ahead – these are the nuts and bolts that will hold your new way of eating together.

GETTING STARTED

You now know how the Gi Diet works, and why it's a great way to lose weight and stay healthy. But you may be wondering what to do first.

Well, let me suggest that you proceed in the following manner.

Note: Before starting any major change in your eating patterns, make sure you check with your doctor.

Charting your progress

Before you do anything else, get your vital statistics on record. Measuring progress is a great motivator. You will find a photocopyable Weight and Waist Log sheet on page 156 to keep in the bathroom and record your weekly progress.

There are two key measurements. The first is weight. Always weigh yourself at the same time of day, because a meal or bowel movement can throw out your weight by a couple of pounds. First thing in the morning, before you eat breakfast, is a good time. The other important measurement is your waist. Measure at your natural waistline – usually just above the navel while standing in a relaxed, normal posture.

Record both measurements on the log sheet. I've added a Comments column to the log sheet where you can note how you're feeling, or any unusual events in the past week that might have some bearing on your progress. Weekly weighing and measuring are recommended.

Clear your fridge and cupboards of red-light foods

Take a look in your fridge, freezer and store cupboards. What do you see? Two jars of mayonnaise, some leftover cheddar and a lot of sugar-laden condiments in jars? At this point, they are almost certain to contain some of the foods that are listed in the red-light column of the Gi Diet Food Guide. Now, how are you going to reach your goal with all this temptation at your fingertips? Banish all red-light products from your home. If you're trying to lose weight, and following Phase I of the Gi Diet, you'll need to get rid of the yellow-light products, too. Don't compromise; put them straight into the bin. If they're not around, you won't be tempted to eat or drink them.

If the thought of throwing them in the bin makes you blanch, donate the tinned foods and other non-perishables to the local food bank and give the rest to skinny neighbours. This does not mean the non-Gi converts in your house will end up feeling deprived as this is a healthy way of eating for everyone.

SHOPPING

Once you've gone through your food stores and got rid of anything that's unsuitable for the Gi Diet, you'll need to stock up at home on green-light products.

You'll find you have to go shopping in a whole different way – but don't worry – it's easy if you follow the Gi guidelines. It's a combination of knowing what makes a low-Gi food, and learning what to look for on the label.

If you find a food in the red-light column that you would normally add to your shopping trolley, look at what's listed beside it in the green-light column. There is almost always a wonderful green-light alternative to a red- or yellow-light food. If, for example, you would normally buy a watermelon, which is a red-light food, choose some oranges, nectarines or grapes, or any of the other green-light choices instead. Remember that if you want to look up a specific food rather than a whole category, you can look at the complete Gi Diet Food Guide on pages 137–150).

If you turn to Appendix II, you will find a shopping list to take with you to the supermarket. As I could not hope to cover the thousands of brands available in most supermarkets, I have listed foods by category e.g. oats, not Scots oats. So if in doubt as to which brand is your best choice, you will have to check the labels.

For the most part, the brand doesn't have any bearing on the Gi rating of a particular food anyway. For example, any low-fat cottage cheese (1 per cent), or wholemeal spaghetti, or Dijon mustard is pretty much the same no matter who's made it. The only times I have mentioned brands is for clarification or a particular 'best buy'.

After a couple of trips, selecting the right products will become second nature.

When comparing brands, here are some guidelines to help you make the best choice.

WHAT TO LOOK FOR ON THE LABEL

NUTRITION INFORMATION

Typical Values per ½ packet:	
Energy	1237kJ/298kcal
Protein	8.9g
Carbohydrate	17.5g (of which sugars 4.2g)
Fat	21.3g (of which saturates 4.4g)
Fibre	1.6g
Sodium	0.1g.
Typical values per 100g:	
Energy	2474kJ/595kcal
Protein	17.8g
Carbohydrate	35.0g (of which sugars 8.4g)
Fat	42.6g (of which saturates 8.8g)
Fibre	3.2g; Sodium 0.2g.

As well as the calorie, fat and fibre levels, there are other things to consider when reading the label.

1. Serving size
Is this realistic, or is the manufacturer lowering it (often the case with cereals) so the calorie and fat totals in particular look better (i.e. less calorific) than their rival brands? When comparing one brand with another, make sure you are comparing the same serving sizes.

2. Calories
The product with the least amount of calories is obviously the best choice.

3. Fat
Choose the product with the least amount of fat, particularly saturated (bad) fat and trans fats. In fact, you should avoid any product that contains trans fat (usually called hydrogenated or partially hydrogenated on the label) – the worst kind of fat for your health.

Also, look for a minimum ratio of 3g of poly- or monounsaturated fat to each gram of saturated fat.

4. Protein
The higher the protein level the better. Protein acts as a brake on the digestive system, thereby lowering the Gi rating of the food.

5. Fibre
Remember, fibre, like protein, significantly lowers the Gi rating, so the product with the higher fibre content is the best choice, whether that fibre is the soluble or insoluble type. Look for a minimum of 4–5g of fibre per serving.

The first is the amount of fibre in the food. Put simply, fibre provides low-calorie filler. High-fibre foods do double duty, in fact, by literally filling up your stomach so that you feel satiated; and by taking much longer to break down in your body, so the digestive process is slowed and the food stays with you longer. And all this helps you to lose weight.

There are two forms of fibre: soluble and insoluble.

Soluble fibre is the kind that's good for your heart. It's found in foods like oats, beans, lentils, barley and many fruits, and has been shown to lower blood cholesterol levels.

Insoluble fibre is the kind that helps your digestive system. It's important for normal bowel function and is typically found in wholemeal breads, other wholegrains, cereals and most vegetables.

6. Sugar
Most green-light foods are low in sugar. Try to avoid products that contain added sugar. Choose the ones with sugar substitutes or none at all.

Watch for products that advertise themselves as 'low fat', despite quietly bumping up the sugar content to make up for any perceived lost taste. Yoghurts and cereals are good examples of this.

Sugars are sometimes listed as dextrose, glucose, fructose or sucrose – regardless of the form, it's sugar.

7. Sodium (salt)
Look for lower sodium and salt levels. Sodium (salt) is linked with high blood pressure, and this, especially combined with excess weight, moves you up to the front of the risk line for heart disease and stroke. Salt also increases water retention, which doesn't help when you are trying to lose weight, and contributes to premenstrual bloating in women.

So, low-sodium products are preferable, because there is hidden salt in many processed products.

The recommended maximum intake of sodium in the UK is 2,400mg (equivalent to a maximum 6g salt), although many authorities, particularly in the UK, are pushing for a reduction to 1,500 mg (4g salt). The current average consumption is 3,600mg sodium (9g salt). Although this is an improvement from the 3,800mg sodium (9.5g salt) we ate in 2001, it still goes without saying that most of us could stand to cut back on salt.

If you have a BMI of over 30 and have any blood pressure, circulation or heart problems, you need to be even more vigilant about seeking out low-sodium brands. We get most of our sodium from manufactured goods, and canned products such as soups are often high in sodium, as are many fast foods.

Label-reading summary

The best green-light buy is:
- Lower in calories
- Lower in fat, particularly saturated fat
- Higher in fibre
- Lower in sugar
- Lower in sodium

A WHISTLE-STOP SUPERMARKET TOUR

The fruit and vegetable aisle

Vegetables and fruit are the cornerstone of the Gi Diet. They are generally low Gi and high in fibre, nutrients, vitamins and minerals. (Cooking them raises their Gi and reduces their nutrient content, so use as little water as possible and cook only until they are just tender – or try eating them raw.)

You'll find that you're buying considerably more fruit and vegetables than previously, so be a little daring and try some varieties that are new to you. There's a wonderful world of fresh and frozen produce just waiting for you to enjoy!

Note: frozen fruits and vegetables have the same nutritional value as fresh.

The deli counter

Most processed meats are high in unhealthy fat, sodium and sodium nitrates, and are therefore red-light. There are, however, a few yellow- and green-light options.

Cheese, too, is pretty much a diet villain, since it's high in saturated fats. However, for flavour, small amounts of strong-flavoured cheeses such as mature Cheddar, feta and Parmesan can be used sparingly, sprinkled on salads, omelettes and pasta.

The dairy section

Low-fat dairy products are a Gi Diet staple. They're rich in protein, calcium and vitamin D. Regular dairy products contain a high amount of saturated fat and are therefore red-light. If you are lactose intolerant, low-fat soya products are an excellent alternative – just make sure they aren't laden with sugar.

The fish counter

All fish and shellfish (so long as they're not breaded or battered) are green-light and provide a wide variety of wonderful meals. Some people are under the mistaken belief that oily fish, such as salmon, tuna and mackerel, isn't good for you. In fact, oily fish is rich in omega-3 and is therefore extremely beneficial for heart health.

The meat counter

Meat always contains some fat, but some cuts have far less than others. Simply trimming visible fat can reduce the overall amount by an average of 50 per cent. Remember to keep the serving size to 4 ounces (110g), which is about the size of the palm of your hand.

Skinless chicken or turkey breast is really the benchmark for low-fat protein. Dark meat, or thighs and legs, duck and goose are higher in saturated fat.

The chiller cabinet

Soya-based foods such as tofu are high in protein, low in saturated fat and good for a healthy heart. Many supermarkets sell textured vegetable protein (TVP) and it is used to make veggie burgers or breakfast sausages and other products. It's an excellent choice whether you're vegetarian or not. Quorn is also a popular alternative.

The frozen food section

Almost all the prepared meals you find in the frozen food section of your supermarket are red-light because of the ingredients used and the way in which they've been processed. Still, the freezer section is a great source of green-light convenience foods such as frozen vegetables and fruit, fish and green-light desserts. Make sure the vegetables aren't in a butter, cream or cheese sauce – that's definitely red-light!

The bakery

The bakery section provides a good illustration of how tricky it can sometimes be to distinguish green-light products from red-light. Let's look at
bread, for example. We know that white bread is red-light, since it spikes
glucose levels in your bloodstream, releasing insulin, which stores the
glucose as fat. The green-light alternative is wholegrain bread, but many
of the healthy-looking seven-grain loaves out there are not exactly what
they seem. Some of them list 'enriched white flour' or 'unbleached flour' in
the ingredients list and this puts a red flashing light over them. The first ingredient listed on bread should always be '100% wholemeal flour' or '100%
wholegrain flour'. If 'stone-ground' is mentioned, even better. There should
also be a minimum of 2.5–3.0 grams of fibre per slice.

Because most people are in the habit of eating white bread, which has
been stripped of most of its nutrients, they are unused to wholegrain
breads. But once you give them a chance, I think you'll find green-light
breads far tastier than bland white loaves.

While you're in the bakery section, remember that anything made primarily of bleached white flour – which has one of the highest Gi ratings of any
food – is red-light. And all the desserts you'll find in the bakery section are
red-light, because of the white flour and sugar in them. But don't despair
– you can make your own delectable desserts at home, using the recipes in
this book.

The tinned beans and vegetable aisle

Beans, or legumes, are the perfect green-light food. They are rich in protein
and fibre and low in fat. Tinned beans are more convenient than dried beans,
but the canning process significantly raises their Gi rating – sometimes up to
50 per cent.

Likewise, with vegetables. It is always preferable to buy fresh or frozen
vegetables rather than tinned.

The pasta and sauces aisle

Most pasta is green-light, and wholemeal pasta is even more so. Make
sure that you always slightly undercook pasta – until it's just al dente, as
the Italians say – and watch the serving size (40g [1½oz] dry weight per
serving).

Choose low-sugar pasta sauces made primarily of tomatoes. Tomato sauce
happens to be rich in lycopene, which has been shown to reduce the risk
of certain cancers, especially prostate cancer. Sauces with cream and/or
cheese are, of course, red-light.

The grains aisle

Whole grains with all the nutrition and fibre intact are usually green-light. With rice, it all depends on the variety, because some contain a starch, amylase, that breaks down slowly. Brown and basmati rice are best.

The cooking oil, vinegar, salad dressing and pickles aisle

Choosing the right oil to use in cooking and on salads is critical to the health of your heart. Saturated and hydrogenated oils (which contain trans fats) are dangerous and should be avoided. Vegetable and olive oils get the green light.

Because acid tends to reduce the Gi rating of a meal – it slows the digestive process – vinegars and vinaigrettes are great additions. Dressings should always be low fat, but be careful of sugar levels. Sometimes producers will raise the sugar level as they reduce the oil to improve flavour. Be sure to check labels and compare low-fat brands.

The snacks aisle

Unfortunately, the snacks aisle at the supermarket is a minefield of red-light temptation. However, you should still be eating three snacks a day – green-light ones of course.

You'll find plenty of green-light snack ideas in the Menu Plan section of this book, and some recipes, too. But is there anything you can buy from the supermarket? Perhaps surprisingly, cereal bars are absolutely red-light – they're full of sugar. If you buy food bars, make sure they contain 20–30g of carbohydrates, 12–15g of protein and 5g of fat. A good green-light choice is Slim-Fast (half a bar per serving).

The home-baking ingredients aisle

Most dried fruit is very high in sugar and therefore red-light. However, there are some yellow-light choices (see Appendix I). Nuts are an excellent source of good fats and protein and green-light nuts contain even more monounsaturated fat (the best kind) than the others. Remember, though, that all nuts are calorie dense and so must be eaten in limited quantities, about eight to twelve per serving. It's just too easy to unconsciously consume a whole bowl of nuts in front of the television, but this quantity would equal your total calorie needs for an entire day!

Although you can't eat ready-made baked goods from the supermarket when you're on the Gi Diet, you can bake your own sweet treats using my recipes. They call for sugar substitutes rather than sugar, honey or treacle. My favourite brand of sweetener is Splenda®, which is derived from sugar but doesn't have the calories. A small amount of dried fruit is acceptable for baking.

The breakfast cereals aisle

Of course, as I've already said, the king of breakfast foods is old-fashioned porridge – the large flake kind, not instant or quick oats. Most cereals on the market are red-light as they're made from highly processed grains that lack both nutrition and fibre. Beware of those so-called healthy or natural granola-types of cereal, because they too are usually low in fibre and high in sugar.

What you should be looking for are cereals that have at least 10g of fibre per serving. They can be dressed up with nuts, fruit and yoghurt.

The beverages aisle

You need up to eight glasses of liquid a day to keep your body hydrated and healthy. Drinks with caffeine tend to stimulate the appetite and so are red-light. The exception is tea, which has far less caffeine than either coffee or soft drinks.

> **CAUTION:** Don't go food shopping with an empty stomach or you'll end up buying items that don't belong to the Gi Diet! Have a healthy green-light snack before you go out.

PERFECT PORTIONS

You can, with a few exceptions (marked with asterisks on the charts), eat as much of the green-light foods as you like (within reason, of course; five heads of cabbage might be going too far). See the table on page 35 for a list of recommended green-light servings. This isn't a deprivation diet. While following the Gi Diet, you should be eating three meals and three snacks daily. Don't leave your digestive system with nothing to do. The saying, 'The devil finds work for idle hands,' might also be applied to your stomach. If your digestive system is busy processing food and steadily supplying energy to your brain, it won't be sending you looking for high-calorie snacks.

Each meal and snack should contain, if possible, a combination of green-light protein, carbohydrates – especially fruit and vegetables – and fats. An easy way to visualise what size these portions should be is to imagine your plate divided into three sections: half the plate should be covered with vegetables; one quarter should contain protein, such as lean meats, seafood, eggs or, if vegetarian, tofu or soya-based foods; and the last quarter should contain a green-light serving of rice, pasta or potatoes.

Here is how your Gi Diet green-light plate should look:

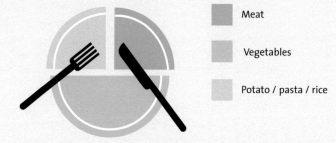

Meat

Vegetables

Potato / pasta / rice

It's important that you spread your daily calorie intake evenly throughout the day. I know that many people make a habit of skipping breakfast in the morning, but this is a big mistake. People who miss breakfast leave their stomachs empty from dinner to lunch the next day, often more than sixteen hours! No wonder they overeat at lunch and then look for a sugar fix mid-afternoon as they run out of steam.

Also, try to consume approximately the same amount of food at each principal meal. If you eat a tiny breakfast and then a tiny lunch, you'll feel so hungry by dinner time that you won't be able to stop yourself from overeating.

Vegetables and fruit, most of which are low-calorie and low-Gi, form the basis of the Gi Diet. Most official sources have traditionally suggested that grains should be the largest component of your diet, followed by vegetables and fruit. But by giving grains priority, they are promoting the leading cause of overweight and obesity. Recently, many of these official sources, including the UK government, have begun to promote vegetables and fruits as the basis of a healthy diet, rather than grains, which is exactly what the Gi Diet recommends.

Recommended green-light servings:	
Green-light breads (these have at least 2.5–3g fibre per slice)	1 slice
Green-light cereals	50g (1³⁄₄oz)
Green-light nuts	8–10
Margarine (non-hydrogenated, light)	2 tsp
Meat, fish, poultry (about the size of a pack of cards)	120g (4oz)
Olive/vegetable oil	1 tsp
Olives	4–5
Pasta (uncooked)	40g (1¹⁄₂oz)
Potatoes (new, boiled)	2–3
Rice: basmati, brown, long-grain (uncooked)	50g (2oz)

BREAKFAST

Breakfast is the first thing you eat after your night-long 'fast' of 12 hours or more, and it launches you into your workday. The right sort of breakfast will help you avoid the need to grab a coffee and a Danish pastry as soon as you hit the office; it will send you off feeling light, energetic and well fed. And it doesn't mean you have to set the alarm any earlier either. If you have time to read the paper or feed the cat, you have time to prepare and eat a green-light breakfast.

You should include some green-light carbohydrates, protein and fat. You'll find a chart of the most common breakfast foods in each light category later in this chapter, and a complete listing of green-, yellow- and red-light foods in Appendix I.

Let's take a closer look at some of the usual breakfast choices.

Cereals

My favourite breakfast of all time is good old-fashioned porridge oats (not the instant type in packets but the large-flake, slow-cooking kind). They're starting to serve it in the smartest hotels now. Not only is large-flake oatmeal low Gi, but it's also low-calorie and has been shown to lower cholesterol. Yes, you have to cook it, but this takes about three minutes or so in the microwave. You can also endlessly vary the flavour by adding non-fat, sugar-free, fruit-flavoured yoghurt, or unsweetened apple sauce/purée, fruit, or sliced almonds. It's also just fine with nothing but milk on it. I probably receive more emails about people's delight in rediscovering por-ridge than about any other food or meal.

Aside from porridge, go for the high-fibre products that have at least 10 grams of fibre per serving. Most cold cereals contain hidden or not-so-hidden sugars, and are red-light. Oat bran is an excellent choice. If you want to, you can liven your cereal up with fresh, canned or frozen fruits, a few nuts or some fruit yoghurt (fat-free, with sweetener).

Toast

Go ahead, but no more than one slice per meal. Choose bread that has at least 2.5–3g of fibre per slice. (Note: Many breads quote a two-slice serving, which should equal 5–6g per serving.) The best choice is 100% stone-ground wholemeal bread. 'Stone-ground' means the flour has been ground with stones rather than steel rollers, resulting in a coarser grind and a lower Gi rating. White bread, cracked wheat or anything else made with white flour is red-light.

Spreads

Butter is out. It's very high in saturated fat, and despite the protestations of the dairy industries, it's not good for your waistline or your health. Yes, it does make things taste good – that's what fat does best! The latest premium brands of non-hydrogenated soft margarine are acceptable and the light versions even more so, but still use them sparingly.

For jams, look for the 'extra fruit/no sugar added' varieties. Fruit, not sugar, should be the first ingredient listed. They taste great and don't have the calories of the usual commercial jams.

Eggs

Whole eggs are a yellow-light food, so, in Phase I, use egg whites where possible. Otherwise, use omega-3 whole eggs (e.g. Columbus) but limit the number to seven per week. Unless you have a medical cholesterol problem, you may eat as many as you wish in Phase II.

Bacon

Sorry, but regular bacon is a red-light food because of its high saturated-fat content. However, there are tasty green-light alternatives, such as back bacon, turkey bacon and lean ham.

Dairy

Low-fat dairy products are an ideal green-light choice and an excellent source of protein in the morning. I always have a glass of skimmed milk with breakfast. Try moving down from semi-skimmed to skimmed in stages. I find that semi-skimmed tastes like cream now!

Low- or non-fat yoghurt that contains sweetener, such as Splenda®, instead of sugar is ideal for breakfast, dessert or a snack, either by itself or added to fruits or cereals.

Low-fat cottage cheese is also a top-rated green-light source of protein. Or you can make a low-fat soft-cheese spread by letting yoghurt drain in cheesecloth overnight in the refrigerator.

Regular, full-fat dairy products, including whole milk and cream, cheese and butter are loaded with saturated fat and calories, and should be avoided completely.

Juice/fruit

Always eat the fruit rather than drink its juice! Juice is a processed product that is more rapidly digested than the parent fruit. To illustrate the point, diabetics who run into an insulin crisis and are in a state of hypoglycaemia (low blood sugar) are usually given orange juice because it's such a fast way to get glucose into the bloodstream.

Coffee and tea

This is the toughest one. The trouble with coffee is caffeine. It's not a health problem in itself, but it does stimulate the production of insulin. That's part of the 'buzz' we go looking for from coffee. But insulin reduces blood-sugar levels, which then increases your appetite. Have you ever or-dered a large coffee from Starbucks and then felt positively shaky an hour later? That's your blood sugar hitting bottom. You cure it by eating – which is when a muffin seems like the only choice.

This caffeine cycle is not helpful when you are trying to keep your appetite stable and under control. So, in Phase I, try to cut out coffee altogether. As unpleasant as it is, caffeine withdrawal is over in a day or two. First, cut down on quantity, from medium to small; then try a half-caffeinated, half- decaffeinated blend. Or you can limit yourself to decaffeinated coffee – some taste as good as the real thing. Even better, switch to tea. It has only about a third of the caffeine of coffee, and black tea has health benefits as well: it's rich in antioxidants, and beneficial for heart health and reducing the risk of dementias. Green tea is also considered an anti-carcinogen. (My 97-year-old mother and her tea-drinking cronies are living proof!) Herbal teas, such as peppermint, chamomile and other blends, are fine, too, as long as they contain no caffeine. But if coffee is going to be a deal breaker, then go ahead, have one cup a day, but not a double espresso. If you take milk and sugar, make it skimmed milk and a sweetener such as Splenda®.

PROTEIN	Red	Yellow	Green
Meat, poultry and eggs	Regular bacon Sausages Whole regular eggs	Turkey bacon Whole omega-3 eggs	Back bacon Lean deli ham Egg whites
Dairy	Cheese Cottage cheese (regular) Cream Milk (whole) Sour cream Yoghurt (regular)	Cream cheese (light) Milk (semi-skimmed) Sour cream (light) Yoghurt (low-fat with sugar)	Buttermilk Cheese (fat-free) Cottage cheese (low-fat or fat-free) Fruit yoghurt (non-fat with sugar substitute) Milk (skimmed) Soya milk (plain, low-fat)
CARBOHYDRATES			
Cereals	All cold cereals except those listed as amber- or green-light Granola Muesli (commercial)	Shredded wheat	All-Bran Oat Bran Porridge (traditional large-flake e.g. Jordan's)
Breads/grains	Bagels Baguettes Biscuits Doughnuts Muffins Pancakes Waffles White bread	Crispbreads (with fibre) Wholemeal breads*	100% stone-ground whole-meal bread* Crispbreads (with fibre, e.g. Ryvita High Fibre) Wholemeal high-fibre breads (2.5–3g fibre per slice)*

Fruits	Apple purée (containing sugar) Tinned fruit in syrup Melons Most dried fruit	Apricots (fresh and dried)** Bananas Dried cranberries** Fruit cocktail in juice Kiwi Mango Papaya Pineapple	Apples Berries Cherries Grapefruit Grapes Oranges Peaches Plums
Juices	Fruit drinks Prune Sweetened juices Watermelon	Apple (unsweetened) Grapefruit (unsweetened) Orange (unsweetened) Pear (unsweetened)	Eat the fruit rather than drink its juice
Vegetables	Chips Hash browns		Most vegetables
FATS			
Fats	Butter Hard margarine Peanut butter (regular and light) Tropical oils Vegetable shortening	Most nuts 100% peanut butter Soft margarine (non-hydrogenated) Vegetable oils	Almonds* Hazelnuts* Olive oil* Soft margarine (non-hydrogenated, light)*

* Limit serving size (see page 35).
** For baking, it is OK to use a modest amount of dried apricots or cranberries.

LUNCH

Lunch is the meal most of us eat outside the home. It can also be the most problematic, limited by time, budget and availability considerations. Because meals where we're not in control of what's on the menu can be tricky, I've given 'eating away from home' a chapter of its own – Chapter 5.

Most people lunching at home will have a light and simple meal, such as a soup and salad.

Salads
Salads are almost always green-light but are often short on protein. Make up the shortfall by adding chickpeas or other types of beans, or 110g (4oz) of tuna, salmon, tofu, skinless, cooked chicken breast or other lean meat. Also, watch the dressing, and use only low-fat or fat-free versions.

Soups
In general, commercially tinned soups have a relatively high-Gi rating because of the necessary high temperatures used in the canning process. There are a few green-light brands, such as Baxter's Healthy Choice.

Homemade soups made with green-light ingredients are the best option, and you'll find some recipes in Chapter 7. Beware of all cream-based or puréed-vegetable soups, since they are high in fat and calories, and heavily processed.

Dessert

Always have some fresh fruit for dessert. Pass on other sweet things at lunch time.

Here's a listing of some popular lunchtime foods, divided into their red-, yellow- and green-light categories. For a complete listing of foods, turn to Appendix I.

PROTEIN	Red	Yellow	Green
Meat, poultry fish, eggs and soy	Beef burgers Beef mince (more than 10% fat) Hot dogs Pâté Processed meats Regular bacon Sausages Whole regular eggs	Beef mince (lean) Lamb (lean cuts) Pork (lean cuts) Tofu Turkey bacon Whole omega-3 eggs	All fish and seafood, fresh or frozen (not battered or breaded) or canned in water Beef (lean cuts) Beef mince (extra-lean) Chicken breast (skinless) Egg whites Tofu (low-fat) Turkey breast (skinless) Veal
CARBOHYDRATES			
Breads/grains	Bagels Baguettes Beef burger or hot dog buns Biscuits Cake Crispbreads Croissants Croutons Doughnuts Muffins Noodles Pancakes Pasta filled with cheese or meat Pizza Rice (short-grain, white, instant) Tortillas Waffles	Crispbreads (with fibre) Pitta (wholemeal) Wholemeal breads*	100% stone-ground wholemeal bread* Crispbreads (high-fibre, e.g. Ryvita High Fibre) Pasta (fettuccine, linguine, macaroni, penne, spaghetti) Quinoa Rice (basmati, wild, brown, long-grain) Wholemeal high-fibre breads (2.5–3g fibre per slice)*

Fruits and vegetables	Broad beans Chips Melons Most dried fruit Parsnips Potatoes (mashed or baked) Swede Turnip	Apricots Artichokes Bananas Beetroot Kiwi Mango Papaya Pineapple Potatoes (boiled) Squash Sweet corn Sweet potatoes	Apples Asparagus Aubergine Avocado ('/₄ per serving) Beans (green/runner) Blackberries Broccoli Brussels sprouts Cabbage Carrots Cauliflower Celery Cherries Chilli peppers Courgettes Cucumber Grapefruit Grapes Leeks Lemons Lettuce Mangetout Mushrooms Olives* Onions Oranges (all varieties) Peaches Pears Peas Peppers (green and red) Pickles Plums Potatoes (new, boiled) Radishes Raspberries Rocket Spinach Strawberries Tomatoes
FATS			
Fats	Butter Hard margarine Mayonnaise (regular) Peanut butter (regular and light) Salad dressings (regular) Tropical oils Vegetable shortening	Mayonnaise (light) Most nut 100% peanut butter Salad dressings (light) Soft margarine (non-hydrogenated)	Almonds* Mayonnaise (fat-free) Olive oil* Salad dressings (low-fat, low-sugar) Soft margarine (non-hydrogenated, light)*
SOUPS			
Soups	All cream-based soups Tinned black bean Tinned green pea Tinned puréed vegetable Tinned split pea	Tinned chicken noodle Tinned lentil Tinned tomato	Chunky bean and vegetable soups (e.g. Baxter's Healthy Choice)

* Limit serving size (see page 35).

DINNER

The typical British dinner comprises three things: meat or fish; potato, pasta or rice; and vegetables. Together, these foods provide an assortment of carbohydrates, proteins and fats, along with other minerals and vitamins essential to our health.

But dinner can be a danger time. At the end of the day, we may have more time to eat – and to overeat. And the fatigue that arrives towards the end of the day is an encouragement to eat too much. There's also a tradition of eating more at dinner. Family dinners can present challenges, too: sometimes the designated cook has to feed two shifts – children first, then late-arriving partners. This means more time in the kitchen and more time waiting, making it tempting to graze and snack.

Protein

This part of your dinner should cover no more than one-quarter of your plate (assuming you don't use huge plates!). A serving size should be 110g (4oz). A portion of meat, poultry or fish should fit into the palm of your hand and be about as thick. Another good visual is a pack of cards.

Red meat

This is allowed, but most red meat contains saturated fat. However, there are a few ways to minimise the fat:

• Buy only low-fat meats such as top round beef. For hamburgers or spaghetti sauces, buy extra-lean minced beef, or buy lean cuts and mince it yourself. Veal or pork tenderloin are low-fat, too. As for juicy steaks, well, they are juicy because of the fat in them, so they're not a good choice.
• Trim any visible fat. Just 5mm (¼in) of fat can double the total amount of fat in the meat.
• Grilling allows the excess fat from the meat to drain off. (Try a George Foreman-style fat-draining electric grill.)
• For cooking on the hob, use a non-stick pan, with a vegetable-oil spray, rather than try to fry with a teaspoon of oil. The spray goes further.

Poultry

Chicken and turkey breast – without the skin – are excellent green-light choices. In the yellow-light category are skinless thighs, wings and legs, which are higher in fat.

Seafood

Always a good green-light choice, so long as it's not breaded or battered. Although certain fish such as salmon and tuna have a relatively high oil content, fish oil is beneficial to your heart health. Prawns and squid are fine, too. Fish and chips, alas, are out.

VEGETARIANS

If you are a non-meat-eater and want to lose weight, the Gi Diet is the programme for you. All you have to do is continue to substitute vegetable protein for animal protein – something you've been doing all along. However, because most vegetable-protein sources, such as beans, are encased in fibre, your digestive system may not be getting the maximum protein benefit. So try to add some easily digestible protein boosters such as tofu and soya-protein powder to your meals.

Beans (legumes)

Beans are a good source of fibre, low-fat protein, and complex carbs that deliver nutrients while taking their time going through the digestive system. And they are a snap to incorporate into salads and soups to add your quotient of protein. Chickpeas, flageolet beans, haricot beans, black beans, kidney beans – a bean for every day of the week. And don't forget lentils!

But watch out for tinned baked beans and sausages – they're high in sugar and fat. And avoid tinned bean soups, where the processing has increased the overall Gi rating.

You will find several delicious recipes using beans in Chapter 7.

Soya (tofu)

You don't have to be vegetarian to enjoy soya, which is low in saturated fat and an excellent source of protein. While tofu is not a thriller on its own, it 'cooks up well', and takes on the flavours of whatever dishes it is added to. Seasoned tofu scrambles, for instance, are a good substitute for scrambled eggs. Choose soft (or 'silken') tofu, which can contain up to a third less fat than the firm variety.

Textured vegetable protein (TVP)

TVP is a soya alternative to meat that looks a lot like minced beef, and can be used in the same ways – in lasagne, chilli, stir-fry and spaghetti sauce. It's quite tasty and delivers the texture of meat. You can buy it chilled, frozen or dried. Our middle son, a vegetarian who has since left the nest, put us on to this adaptable product.

Starchy carbohydrates

These are the ones that veteran dieters have been conditioned to avoid. But they are fine as long as they only cover one-quarter of the plate.

Potatoes

The Gi ratings of potatoes vary from high to moderate, depending on how they are cooked. Boiled new potatoes are the only kind you should eat, two or three at a sitting. All other choices, especially baked potatoes, chips or French fries, are red-light. Incidentally, although sweet potatoes are not technically potatoes, they are a good lower-Gi food. But since they tend to come in larger sizes, I suggest you save these for Phase II.

Pasta

Though most pastas have a moderate-Gi rating and are low in fat, they have become a villain in weight control. That's because we tend to eat portions that are too large. Italians quite rightly view pasta as an appetiser or side dish, while we make it a main course with sauce and a few slivers of meat. Pasta should only make up a quarter of your meal (about 40g [1½oz] uncooked). Use whole-wheat or protein-enriched pasta and stay away from cream-based sauces.

And remember to undercook it a little so that it is slightly firm to the bite (al dente).

Rice

Rice has a broad Gi range. The low ones are basmati, wild, brown and long grain because they contain a starch, called amylose, that breaks down more slowly than that of other rices. Serving size is critical, too. Allow 50 grams (1¾oz) of dry rice per serving.

Vegetables/salad

Eat green-light vegetables and salad to your heart's content – here you can put the scales away. Serve two or three varieties of vegetables at every dinner as well as a salad – they should be the backbone of your meal. Greens such as rocket or baby spinach come conveniently pre-washed in bags. Frozen bags of mixed vegetables are inexpensive and convenient; you can even toss the veggies into a saucepan, add tomato juice with a dollop of salsa and you have a quick vegetable soup.

Experiment with something you've never had before. Baby pak choi is delicious grilled, and rapini, a dark-green vegetable that looks like broccoli with more leaves, is a nice change. The dark, curly green vegetables such as kale have a strong taste and are full of good things, including folic acid.

DESSERTS

There is a broad range of low-Gi, low-calorie green-light desserts that taste great and are good for you. Virtually any fruit qualifies and there's always low-fat, sugar-free dairy products (including low-fat, sugar-free ice cream). You'll also find some great recipes in this book.

With the pitfalls of dinner in mind, here is our traffic-light chart listing popular dinnertime foods. Remember that you can find a full list of foods in Appendix I.

PROTEIN	Red	Yellow	Green
Meat, poultry fish and eggs	Beef burgers Beef mince (more than 10% fat) Breaded fish and seafood Fish tinned in oil Hot dogs Processed meats Sausages Sushi Whole regular eggs	Beef mince (lean) Lamb (lean cuts) Pork (lean cuts) Whole omega-3 eggs	All fish and seafood, fresh or frozen (not battered, breaded or tinned in oil) Beef (lean cuts) Beef mince (extra-lean) Chicken breast (skinless) Egg whites Lean deli ham Turkey breast (skinless) Veal
Dairy	Cheese Cottage cheese (regular) Milk (whole) Soured cream Yoghurt (regular)	Cheese (low-fat) Milk (semi-skimmed) Soured cream (light) Yoghurt (low-fat)	Cheese (fat-free) Cottage cheese (fat-free) Fruit yoghurt (non-fat with sugar substitute) Soya milk (plain, low-fat)
CARBOHYDRATES			
Breads/grains	Bagels Baguettes Biscuits Cake Croissants Doughnuts Muffins Noodles Pasta filled with cheese or meat Pizza Rice (short-grain, white, instant) Tortillas	Pitta (wholemeal) Wholemeal breads*	100% stone-ground wholemeal bread* Pasta (fettuccine, linguine, macaroni, penne, spaghetti)* Quinoa Rice (basmati, wild, brown, long-grain) Wholemeal high-fibre breads (2.5–3g fibre per slice)*
Fruits and vegetables	Broad beans Chips Melons Most dried fruit Parsnips Potatoes (mashed or baked) Swede Turnip	Apricots Bananas Beetroot Kiwi Mango Papaya Pineapple Pomegranates	Apples Asparagus Aubergine Avocado (¼ per serving) Beans (green/runner) Blackberries Broccoli **Continues on next page →**

Fruits and vegetables		Potatoes (boiled) Squash Sweet corn Sweet potatoes	Brussels sprouts Cabbage Carrots Cauliflower Celery Cherries Chilli peppers Courgettes Cucumber Grapefruit Grapes Leeks Lemons Lettuce Mangetout Mushrooms Olives* Onions Oranges (all varieties) Peaches Pears Peas Peppers (green and red) Pickles Plums Potatoes (new, boiled) Radishes Raspberries Rocket Spinach Strawberries Tomatoes
FATS			
Fats	Butter Hard margarine Mayonnaise (regular) Peanut butter (regular and light) Salad dressings (regular) Tropical oils	Mayonnaise (light) Most nuts 100% peanut butter Salad dressings (light) Soft margarine (non-hydrogenated) Vegetable oils Walnuts	Almonds* Mayonnaise (fat free) Olive oil* Pistachios Salad dressings (low fat, low sugar) Soft margarine (non-hydrogenated, light)*
SOUPS			
Soups	All cream-based soups Tinned black bean Tinned green pea Tinned puréed vegetable Tinned split pea	Tinned chicken noodle Tinned lentil Tinned tomato	Chunky bean and vegetable soups (e.g. Baxter's Healthy Choice) Homemade soups with green-light ingredients

* Limit serving size (see page 35).

SNACKS

I can't stress enough how important it is to have three snacks every day. Three snacks – mid-morning, mid-afternoon and before bed – will keep your digestive system busy, and your energy levels up. Snacks play a critical role between meals by giving you a boost when you most need it. Make them balanced; for example, a piece of fruit with a few nuts or cottage cheese with celery sticks.

If you're on the move, another convenient snack is half an energy bar. Choose 50- to 65-gram bars that have around 200 calories each with 20 to 30 grams of carbohydrates, 12 to 15 grams of protein and 5 grams of fat. In the UK, these are sometimes hard to find. Check your local sports-equipment or health-food shop. Most so-called nutrition bars found in supermarkets are high Gi, high-calorie, and contain lots of quick-fix carbs, so check the labels carefully. Slim-Fast is a good choice.

Many snacks and desserts are labelled 'low-fat' or 'sugar-free', but they aren't necessarily green-light. Sugar-free instant puddings or 'low-fat' muffins are still high Gi because they contain highly processed grains.

Here's a list of popular snack foods, arranged by Gi traffic-light colours.

SNACKS	Red	Yellow	Green
	Bagels	Bananas	Almonds**
	Biscuits	Dark chocolate (70% cocoa)	Apple sauce (unsweetened)
	Chips	Ice cream (low-fat)	Cottage cheese (fat free)
	Crackers	Most nuts	Extra-low-fat cheese (e.g. Laughing Cow Light, Boursin Light)
	Crisps	Popcorn (air-popped)	
	Doughnuts		Food bars*
	Flavoured jelly (all varieties)		Fruit yoghurt (non-fat with sugar substitute)
	Ice cream		Hazelnuts**
	Muffins		Homemade green-light snacks (see pages 73–75)
	Popcorn (regular)		Ice cream (low-fat and no added sugar)
	Pretzels		
	Puddings		Most fresh fruit
	Raisins		Most fresh vegetables
	Rice cakes		Peaches tinned in juice or water
	Sorbet		Pears tinned in juice or water
	Tortilla chips		Pickles
	Trail mix		Pumpkin seeds
	Sweets		Sugar-free sweets
	White bread		Sunflower seeds

* 180–225 calorie bars, e.g. Slim-Fast; ½ bar per serving.

** Limit serving size (see page 35).

DRINKS

Because liquids don't trip our satiety mechanisms, it's a waste to take in calories through them. And many beverages are high-calorie. Fruit juice, for example, is a processed product and has a much higher Gi than the fruit or vegetable it is made from. A glass of orange juice contains nearly two and a half times the calories of a fresh orange. So, eat the fruit or vegetable rather than drink its juice. That way, you'll get all the benefits of its nutrients and fibre while consuming fewer calories. The Gi value will be lower, too.

As well, we should stay away from any beverage that contains added sugar or caffeine. As I explained earlier, caffeine stimulates insulin, which leads to us feeling hungry.

That said, fluids are an important part of any diet and I'm sure you're familiar with the eight-glasses-a-day prescription. Personally, I find this a bit steep. But I do try to drink a glass of water before each meal and snack. Other than to stay hydrated, I do this for two reasons: one, having your stomach partly filled with liquid before the meal means you will feel full more quickly, thus reducing the temptation to overeat; two, you won't be tempted to wash down your food before it's been sufficiently chewed.

The following are your best green-light choices:

Water
Water is definitely the best beverage choice because it doesn't contain any calories. Seventy per cent of our body consists of water, which is needed for digestion, circulation, regulation of body temperature, lubrication of joints and healthy skin. We can live for weeks without food, but we can only survive a few days without water.

Coffee
If you can, it's best to stick with decaffeinated coffee. Never add sugar (sweetener is fine) and use only semi-skimmed or skimmed milk.

Tea
Both black and green teas have considerably less caffeine than coffee and also contain antioxidants that are beneficial to your heart health, and help prevent Alzheimer's. Two cups of tea have the same amount of antioxidants as seven cups of orange juice or twenty of apple juice! So, tea in moderation is fine, but use a sweetener if you normally add sugar, and have skimmed milk.

Try different varieties – Darjeeling, Earl Grey, English Breakfast or the spicy chai teas. Herbal teas are also an option, although they lack the flavonoids. Iced tea is acceptable if it's sugar-free.

Soft drinks

People often treat soft drinks or fruit juices as non-foods, but this is how extra calories slip by us. But if you're used to drinking soft drinks, you can still enjoy them if you buy sugar- and caffeine-free diet drinks.

Skimmed milk

Skimmed milk is virtually fat-free, and since most breakfasts and lunches tend to be protein deficient, drinking skimmed milk is a good way of making up for some of the shortfall.

Soya milk

Soya milk can be an excellent choice, but buyer beware: most soya beverages are not only high in fat, but also have added sugar. Look for soya milk that is low-fat, that has no flavouring like vanilla or chocolate and is sold as 'unsweetened'.

Alcohol

Alcohol is a disaster if you're concerned about your weight. It puts your blood sugar on a roller coaster: you go up and feel great, then come down and start feeling like having another drink, or eating the whole bowl of peanuts, setting you on a cycle of highs and lows.

On the other hand, a little red wine can be beneficial for your heart health and, in Phase II, I encourage you to have a glass of wine with dinner. So you can look forward to that! But, in the meantime, put away the corkscrew and the ice-cube tray because Phase I is an alcohol-free zone.

Here's a list of popular drinks, broken down into their Gi traffic-light colours.

EVERAGES	Red	Yellow	Green
	Chocolate milk mix	Diet soft drinks (caffein-ated)	Bottled water (sparking or still)
	Coffee (regular)	Most unsweetened juice	Decaffeinated coffee
	Coffee whitener	Non-alcoholic beer	Diet soft drinks (without caffeine)
	Evaporated milk	Vegetable juices	Herbal teas
	Fruit crystals		Iced tea (with no added sugar)
	Fruit drinks		Light instant chocolate
	Hot chocolate (regular)		Tea (with or without caffeine)
	Iced tea (regular)		
	Soft drinks (regular)		
	Sport drinks		
	Sweetened condensd milk		
	Sweetened juice		
	Tonic water		

Summary

In Phase I, eat only green-light foods – three meals and three balanced snacks per day.

Drink plenty of fluids, including a 240ml (8fl oz) glass of water with meals and snacks (but no caffeine or alcohol).

Pay attention to portion size: palm of your hand for protein, and a quarter plate for pasta, potatoes or rice. Use common sense and eat moderate amounts.

Don't get discouraged by lapses. If you eat green-light 90% of the time, you'll still be fine.

5 Eating Away from Home

These days, we eat more of our food than ever away from home. Sometimes this can be helpful – when we take a packed lunch to work, we have total control over what goes into it. In other situations, things are trickier. When you have to grab a snack meal away from home, for example, it can be difficult to find the green-light options.

But it is possible, and I'll show you how. You can even find Gi-allowable foods at fast-food restaurants. It's not easy – but you can do it, if you know what to look for.

LUNCH BOXES

Bringing your own lunch to work is the easiest way to eat green-light foods. And if you're a mother or father who already has to pack school lunches, all you have to do is assemble one more, for you. Besides avoiding the temptation of a red-light lunch: it's cheaper, and it gives you downtime at your desk or outside to read or catch up on paperwork.

Sandwiches

It's not surprising that sandwiches are the lunchtime staple. They're portable, easy to make and offer endless variety. They can also be a dietary disaster – high Gi, high in fat and high in calories. But if you follow the suggestions below you can keep your sandwiches green-light:

• Always use 100% stone-ground wholemeal or high-fibre wholegrain bread (2½–3g fibre per slice).
• During Phase I, sandwiches should be served open-faced. Either pack components separately and assemble just before eating or make your sandwich with a 'lettuce lining' that helps keep the bread from getting soggy. Then discard the extra slice (or share it with the birds).
• No regular mayonnaise or butter. Use mustard or hummus instead.
• Include at least 3 vegetables, such as lettuce, tomato, red or green pepper, cucumber, beansprouts or onion.
• Add up to 110g (4oz) of cooked lean meat or fish – roast beef, turkey, prawns or salmon.
• For tuna- or chicken-salad sandwiches, use low-fat mayonnaise or low-fat salad dressing and celery.
• Mix tinned salmon with malt vinegar or fresh lemon.

Lunchtime salads

Preparing salads may seem more labour-intensive than sandwiches, but it doesn't have to be. Invest in a variety of plastic containers so you can pack them easily. Keep a supply of green-light vinaigrette on hand, wash greens ahead of time and store in paper towels in plastic bags. You'll find that creative salads are a good way to use up leftovers with a minimum of fuss.

Salads are often short on protein, so add in chickpeas or other types of beans, or 110g (4oz) of tuna, salmon, tofu, skinless, cooked chicken breast or other lean meat. Also, watch the dressing, and use only low-fat, fat-free versions or vinaigrette.

Pasta salads

Watch the quantity. Use 40g (1½oz) of pasta (dry weight), preferably whole-meal, plus lots of vegetables and 125g (4½oz) of chicken or turkey meat, or fish.

Cottage cheese, fruit and nuts

A fast, easy and inexpensive lunch. Simply mix together 250g (9oz) of low- or fat-free cottage cheese, some fruit and a handful of sliced almonds.

Dessert

If you have time, a fruit yoghurt with a sugar substitute is terrific. (Müller Light is a best buy.) Always eat some fruit. I keep a supply of apples, pears, peaches and grapes, depending on the season, in my office. Stay away from most other desserts.

SANDWICH BARS

Sandwich bars are an excellent alternative to fast-food outlets as they enable you to customise your sandwich and see exactly what is going into it. Here is what to ask for to ensure your sandwich is green-light:

- Wholemeal, stone-ground or granary bread
- Hummus or mustard in lieu of butter, margarine or mayonnaise
- Lean slices of chicken or turkey breast, ham or tuna as the principal filling. Avoid mayonnaise, cheese and bacon bits
- Add lots of vegetables such as tomatoes, avocado, lettuce, salad leaves or onion rings for flavour and nutrition
- Always remove the top slice of bread and eat the sandwich open-faced

Wraps: An increasingly popular alternative to the traditional sandwich is a wrap.

Pitta pockets: Ask if the pitta bread can be split in half. (My lunch counter thinks I'm odd in this regard and insists on giving me the other half in a separate bag to take with me. I've no idea what they expect me to do with it!)

Baguettes: Again ask for wholewheat bread, and eat it open-faced. Avoid cheese and mayonnaise unless they're low-fat.

EATING OUT AT RESTAURANTS

Dining out on the Gi Diet is not difficult these days, since many restaurants have made the switch to olive or vegetable oils and offer more entrées that are grilled rather than fried, breaded or sauced. They also offer a greater variety of vegetables, salads and fish dishes than in the past. All of these changes in the food culture make it easier to dine out the green-light way. Here are my strategies for not going astray.

Starting out
Once seated in the restaurant, drink a glass of water. It will help you feel fuller, and prevent overeating.

Once the basket of rolls or bread has been passed round the table – which you will ignore! – ask the server to remove it. Flatbreads may look thin and diet-ish but, like crackers, they often have hidden trans fats, and they are not low-calorie. Bread rolls are white flour incarnate. The longer that basket sits there, the more tempted you will be to dig in.

Another good tip is, just before you go out, have a small bowl of high-fibre, green-light cold cereal (such as All-Bran) with skimmed milk and sweetener. I often add a couple of spoonfuls of fruit yoghurt. This will take the edge off your appetite and get some fibre into your digestive system, which will help reduce the Gi of your upcoming meal.

Soups and salads
Order a soup or salad first and tell the server you would like this as soon as possible. This will keep you from sitting there hungry while others are filling up on the bread. For soups, go for vegetable- or bean-based, the chunkier the better. Avoid any that are cream-based, such as vichyssoise.

For salads, the golden rule is to keep the dressing on the side. Then you can use a fraction of what the restaurant would normally pour over the greens – and please avoid Caesar salads, which come pre-dressed and often pack as many calories as a burger.

Meat, poultry and fish

If there's a choice between sautéed and grilled, always go for grilled. Sautéeing usually involves oils or butter.

Stick with low-fat cuts of meat or poultry. If necessary, you can remove the skin of poultry, though you should avoid duck in any form, as it is too high in fat. Fish and shellfish are excellent choices but shouldn't be breaded or battered. And remember that servings tend to be generous in restaurants, so eat only 110–175g (4–6oz, the size of a pack of cards) and leave the rest.

As with salads, ask for any sauces to be put on the side.

Potatoes

If you can't get plain, boiled new potatoes when eating out, ask your waiter for double vegetables in lieu of potatoes. After hundreds of requests, I've never been refused.

Desserts and coffee

For dessert, fresh fruit and berries, if available, are your best choice – without the cream or ice cream. Most other choices are a dietary disaster. My advice is to avoid dessert. If a birthday cake is being passed around, share your piece with someone. A couple of forkfuls or so along with your coffee should get you off the hook, with minimal dietary damage!

Only order decaffeinated coffee. Skim-milk decaf cappuccino is our family's favourite choice.

Finally, and perhaps most important, eat slowly. Put your fork down between bites. The stomach can take up to half an hour to let the brain know it feels full. So if you eat quickly, you may be shovelling in more food than you require, till the brain finally says stop. You will also be able to savour your meal for longer.

FOREIGN CUISINES

Chinese

The two things to watch for are the rice and the sauces, especially the sweet ones, which are high in sugar. Rice is usually a problem, as most restaurants use a glutinous high-GI rice whose grains tend to stick together. If you can be assured the rice is either basmati or long-grain and doesn't clump together, then OK, but limit the quantity to a quarter of your plate.

Indian and South Asian

Probably your best choice. Fruit, vegetables, legumes and wholegrains are predominant in Indian cuisine as is basmati/long-grain rice, all of which are green-light choices. A word of warning: do not eat any fried food as it is often deep-fried in 'ghee' (clarified butter), which is high in saturated (bad) fat.

Pasta

Though most pastas range in the moderate-Gi category, some are clearly preferable to others. A rule of thumb is that thicker pastas are better. Pasta is a villain in our obesity problem not because of any issue with pasta itself – it is a low-fat (although high-calorie) product. The problem lies in the quantities we eat.

Because it's difficult when dining out to order a partial plate of pasta, it's best to avoid it completely. If you are able to obtain a side order, then limit the quantity to cover a quarter of the plate and ask for low-fat sauce options. Please, no cream or cheese sauces such as Alfredo. If wholegrain pasta is available, go for it.

FAST FOOD

A few years ago, the idea of getting a green-light meal at a fast-food restaurant was simply laughable. Now, partly due to the threat of legal action and a stagnant market share, the major fast-food chains are finally offering some healthy options. Subway, for instance, has pioneered the move to healthy choices for some time, and it has been reflected in their successful growth with more outlets than McDonald's worldwide.

The fast-food market is a dynamic one, and, hopefully, market pressures are going to be persuading the big players to introduce more healthier options. You may wish to check these restaurants' menus or websites from time to time to see if they have expanded their green-light offerings. Every restaurant usually has nutritional breakdowns available for its menu items, if you ask for them.

Although things are changing in McDonald's land, fast food is still a minefield. Pizza is red-light all the way thanks to its high-Gi crust and the saturated fat in the cheese toppings. Beefburgers are also soaked in saturated fat, as are breaded, deep-fried chicken and fish. And all the trimmings – fries, ketchup, milkshakes and fizzy drinks – are loaded with fat, sugar and calories.

Merely being in the presence of all those tempting burgers, fries and shakes makes your challenges more difficult – so stay away, if at all possible! I can assure you that after a few months eating the Gi way, even the idea of fast food will turn you off. With your face pressed to the window of McDonald's, you'll watch with amazement what the heavyweights are putting away – straight to their waists and hips. That could have been you!

Still, there are a few points of light in this sea of gloom. If your alternatives are limited, here is how you can successfully navigate through this gastronomic minefield.

• **Burgers:** Dispose of the top of the bun and don't order cheese or bacon. Keep it as simple as possible.
• **Fries:** Just DON'T. A medium order of McDonald's fries contains 17g of fat (mostly saturated), about 50% of your total daily allowance.
• **Milkshakes:** DON'T. The saturated fat, sugar and calorie levels are unbelievable.
• **Salads:** The one bright light is the recent introduction of salads at places such as McDonald's and Burger King. These are a good choice, providing you do not apply the whole sachet of dressing, which can double the calorie content of the meal. Pick the low-fat versions. A half of a pouch is quite sufficient for most people. Keep clear of Caesar salads.
• **Other fast-food outlets:** If you go into other fast-food outlets, such as Tesco Express, Sainsbury Local, Marks & Spencer, Benjys etc., steer clear of sandwiches and rolls containing mayonnaise and cheese. Look for wholemeal and high-fibre breads and eat them open-faced.

6 Cooking on the Gi Diet

COOKING

Cooking on the Gi Diet generally means cooking from scratch and avoiding heavily processed foods. But that doesn't mean you have to spend a lot of time in the kitchen. Most of the suggestions in this book can be made in less than thirty minutes.

Good taste is always my primary consideration. Try to use plenty of fresh herbs, delicious spices and ethnic flavours to come up with interesting and fun meals. To turn your own much-loved recipes green light, you'll need to follow four steps:

1) replace red-light ingredients with green
2) replace sugar with sugar substitute
3) use less fat and make sure it's green-light fat
4) add extra fibre to the recipe

You'll find some breakfast recipes for those mornings when you are on the run, as well as some recipes that are more suited for relaxing weekends. Any of the salad and soup recipes can form the basis of a satisfying lunch, and there are plenty of fish and seafood, poultry, meat and vegetarian dishes for dinner. And because this isn't a deprivation diet, there are some delicious recipes for desserts and snacks to enjoy.

To replace sugar in recipes, I've had great success with Splenda® and have found the flavour quite good. Look for the granular type that comes in boxes because it is the easiest to use – you can measure out the amount just like sugar.

Equipment

Non-stick frying pans
When cooking low-fat dishes, it's useful to have a few non-stick pans in various sizes. You only need a minimal amount of oil when using them and food slides right off the pan. Remember that the recommended cooking

heat for non-stick surfaces is no higher than medium-high and that you should use non-abrasive utensils and brushes only. Wash your frying pan with hot soapy water and a nylon brush – do not put it in the dishwasher. Replace your non-stick pans when they begin to show wear and tear.

Grill pan/indoor grill
The tips for caring for your non-stick pans also apply to grill pans and indoor grills. When using them, you only need a light brush or spray of oil. A grill rack keeps the food you are cooking out of the fat and gives that grilled look when you don't have an outdoor barbecue.

Meal planning
If you are a newcomer to the Gi Diet, you may be surprised at the wide-ranging variety of appealing green-light foods. Not only are these green-light foods good for you, but I also happen to think that they are some of the best tasting.

I have tried to adapt meals that are commonly used by most of us, so there is no need to worry about the unfamiliar. These meal ideas not only use green-light foods, but I've also kept the use of fats in cooking to a minimum.

Cutting fat doesn't mean you have to cut flavour or lose that all-important taste sensation:

• Cream can be replaced by yoghurt, yoghurt cheese (see page 86) or cottage cheese.
• Use low-/no-fat mayonnaise in tuna or chicken salads.
• You can still use cheese, especially the strongly flavoured ones, but sprinkle it sparingly as a flavour enhancer only, rather than using it as the prime ingredient.
• Try some new spices and flavoured vinegars.
• Salsa will spice up many foods without adding calories or fat, and ginger adds life to stir-fries.

All of the recipes you will find in this book are straightforward, easy to follow and the ingredients are readily available at your local supermarket.

The following recipes have been selected from other books in the Gi Diet series, and are representative of the many delicious recipes available, particularly in my *Gi Diet Green-light Cookbook* and *Living the Gi Diet*.

BREAKFAST

Porridge (see Homey Oatmeal, page 104) can be endlessly varied by changing the flavour of the fruit yoghurt or adding sliced fruit or berries.

Other excellent and speedy breakfasts you might like to try are Homemade Muesli (see page 82), On-the-run Breakfast (below) or Hot Kasha Cereal (below).

ON-THE-RUN BREAKFAST (1 serving)

Combine:
40g (1½oz) All-Bran/High-Fibre Bran
160g (5½oz) fresh fruit
110gl (4fl oz) cottage cheese (low-fat)
2 tbsp sliced almonds

Have this with 1 slice toast, 2 tsp low-fat non-hydrogenated spread and 1 tbsp reduced-sugar jam, 1 cup decaffeinated coffee or tea.

HOT KASHA CEREAL (4 servings)
This is a good basic hot cereal that is a change from traditional porridge. Stir in some fresh fruit or a few chopped nuts if liked.

180g (6oz) buckwheat grains (kasha)
2 tbsp ground flaxseed
2 tbsp sesame seeds
2 tbsp wheat germ
Pinch of salt
Sugar substitute and ground cinnamon, to taste

1. In a medium saucepan, bring 750ml (1 1/3 pints) water to boil. Stir in the buckwheat, flax, sesame seeds, wheat germ and salt. Return to a simmer and cook for about 12–15 minutes, stirring occasionally. Stir in the sugar substitute and cinnamon to taste. If a thinner consistency is preferred, mix in a little water or skimmed milk.

At weekends when breakfasts (or brunch) can sometimes be a more leisurely meal, omelettes are always welcome. You can vary them by adding any number of fresh vegetables, a little cheese and/or some meat.

OMELETTE (1 serving)

Vegetable oil cooking spray (preferably rapeseed or olive oil)
2–3 omega-3 eggs, beaten (alternatively, use 1 egg and 2 whites if in Phase I of the Gi Diet)
55ml (2fl oz) skimmed milk

1. Spray oil in a small non-stick frying pan, then place it over medium heat. If you're making one of the omelette variations, add the mushrooms, peppers, broccoli and/or onion (depending on which omelette you are making) and sauté until tender, about 5 minutes. Transfer the sautéed vegetables to a plate and cover with aluminium foil to keep warm.

2. Now make the omelette. Beat the eggs with the milk and pour them into the frying pan over medium heat. Cook until the eggs start to firm up then spread the appropriate vegetables, cheese, herbs, beans and/or meat over them. Continue cooking until the eggs are done to your liking.

3. If desired, sprinkle the omelette with hot sauce, chilli powder, red pepper flakes, then serve.

VARIATIONS:
ITALIAN OMELETTE
To the basic omelette recipe, add:
25g (1oz) grated skimmed mozzarella cheese
60g (2½oz) sliced mushrooms
115ml (4floz) tomato purée
Herbs to taste (chopped, fresh or dried herbs such as oregano or basil)

MEXICAN OMELETTE
To the basic omelette recipe, add:
100g (3½oz) mixed canned beans
110g (4oz) chopped red and green peppers
60g (2½oz) sliced mushrooms
Hot sauce or chilli powder to taste (optional)

VEGETARIAN OMELETTE
To the basic omelette recipe, add:
25g (1oz) grated low-fat cheese
50g (2oz) broccoli florets
50g (2oz) sliced mushrooms
50g (2oz) chopped red and green peppers

WESTERN OMELETTE
To the basic omelette recipe, add:
2 slices back bacon, lean deli ham or turkey breast, chopped
1 onion, chopped
110g (4oz) chopped red and green peppers
Herbs to taste

SCRAMBLED EGG VARIATIONS
Make scrambled eggs by stirring the eggs and milk (quantities as in the omelette recipe) as they cook, adding any additional ingredients while the eggs are still soft.

To round off the meal, include some fresh fruit, a glass of skimmed milk or a small carton of fat-free yoghurt with sweetener.

LUNCH

Soup and a sandwich or a salad containing a serving of protein makes a simple and satisfying lunch. Add a piece of green-light fruit and you will be set up for the afternoon. If you can make your own lunch so much the better – you can introduce a lot more variety and you'll know exactly what you are eating.

Sandwiches
The variations are endless – refer to Chapter 5 for some guidelines to make even the humble sandwich a convenient and filling green-light meal.

Wraps
These are growing in popularity and make a good choice in fast-food outlets in particular. Follow the same rules as for sandwiches.

Soups
The soups to go for are the chunky vegetable and barley variety, particularly with beans. Avoid any suggestion of 'cream of ...'

Weekend lunches
At the weekends, have a barbecue lunch – all you need is some meat, poultry or fish and a selection of salads and crusty wholemeal bread – or try Cheese Blintzes (see recipe on page 62).

CHEESE BLINTZES (8 blintzes/4 servings)
In the summer, serve with whatever fresh fruit or berries are in season.

Batter:
60g (2¼oz) wholemeal plain flour
1 tbsp ground flaxseed or wheat germ
Pinch salt
250ml (9fl oz) skimmed milk
2 free-range medium eggs, beaten
1 tsp vanilla extract
1 tbsp rapeseed oil

Filling:
250g tub natural cottage cheese, drained of whey
125g (4½oz) fat-free natural or vanilla yoghurt with sweetener
1 free-range egg
2 tbsp sugar substitute
1 tsp grated lemon zest

1. Make the blintz batter first : In medium bowl, mix together the flour, flaxseed and salt. In another bowl, whisk together the milk, eggs and vanilla, then beat this into the dry ingredients until smooth. Let the batter stand at room temperature for at least 15 minutes, or cover and chill for up to 2 hours.

2. Brush a small non-stick or crêpe pan with just enough oil to lightly coat it. Heat the pan over a medium heat. Pour in about 2 tbsp of the batter, swirling the pan to cover the bottom. Cook the crêpe until firm and slightly golden underneath, about 2 minutes, then flip over and cook the other side for another 30 seconds. Remove to a plate. Repeat with remaining batter, stacking crêpes one on top of the other, you should have at least 8 crêpes. Preheat the oven to 180°C, Gas 4.

3. For the filling: In large bowl, blend together the cottage cheese, yoghurt, egg, sugar substitute and lemon zest.

4. Place the crêpes flat on a work surface. Spoon the filling into the centre of each crêpe. Fold in sides and place blintzes on a lightly greased or baking parchment-paper-lined baking sheet, folded side down. Bake for 25–30 minutes or until heated through. Serve with fresh fruit or berries or a berry sauce from fruit-stuffed French Toast (see recipe on page 91).

CHILLI-LIME TIGER PRAWNS (Makes 4 servings)
Summer barbecue fare.

4 tbsp fresh lime juice
2 hot chillies, seeded and diced
1 tbsp grated lime zest
1 tbsp olive oil
2 tsp chilli powder
500g (1lb 2oz) large raw tiger prawns, shell-on
lime wedges, to serve

1. In a large bowl, beat together the lime juice, chillies, lime zest, olive oil and chilli powder. Stir in the prawns, tossing to coat. Marinate at room temperature for 30 minutes, tossing occasionally.

2. Cook on a medium-high greased grill for 3 minutes per side or until shells are pink. Serve with lime wedges to squeeze over.

Salads
Salads are a valuable addition to meals and a simple way to get fresh vegetables into your diet at lunch and dinner.

EVERYDAY SALAD AND VINAIGRETTE (1 serving)
This is a good basic salad and vinaigrette that you can endlessly vary by using different vegetables, vinegars and herbs.

60g (2½oz) lettuce (such as cos, rocket, watercress, iceberg or mixed leaf)
1 small carrot, shredded
½ pepper (red, yellow or green), sliced
1 plum tomato, cut in wedges
½ sliced cucumber
2 slices of red onion (optional)

In a bowl, toss together the lettuce, carrot, pepper, tomato, cucumber and onion.

VINAIGRETTE (1 serving)

1 tbsp vinegar (such as white or red wine, balsamic, rice or cider) or lemon juice
1 tsp extra-virgin olive oil or rapeseed oil
½ tsp Dijon mustard
Pinch each salt and pepper
Pinch dried or fresh herb of choice (such as thyme, oregano, basil, Italian seasoning, marjoram, mint)

In a small bowl, whisk together the vinegar, oil, mustard, salt, pepper and herb. Pour the dressing over the salad and toss.

FENNEL WALDORF SALAD (4 servings)

This salad is a mix of tastes and textures. Look for leafy, very fresh watercress, preferably in bunches.

3 celery sticks, sliced diagonally
2 apples, (unpeeled) quartered, cored and sliced
1 large navel orange, peeled and segmented
125g (4½oz) red or green seedless grapes
1 small bulb fennel, thinly sliced
1 bunch fresh watercress, trimmed and torn in pieces
40g (1½oz) shelled unsalted pistachios, chopped

Dressing:
4 tbsp low-fat plain yoghurt
2 tbsp reduced-fat mayonnaise
2 tsp rapeseed oil
2 tbsp lemon juice
1 tsp lemon zest
Pinch each sea salt and pepper

1. In large bowl, toss together the celery, apples, orange, grapes and fennel. Make the dressing: In a small bowl, whisk together the yoghurt, mayonnaise, oil, lemon juice, lemon zest and seasoning.

2. Pour the dressing over the fruit and vegetables and toss to coat. Just before serving, toss with the watercress and pistachios.

ESCAROLE AND BERRY SALAD WITH HERB AND LEMON VINAIGRETTE AND BLUE CHEESE (4-6 servings)

Choose escarole with tender, light-green leaves. The dark leaves can be quite bitter.

1 head escarole or curly leaf lettuce, shredded
60g (2¼oz) fresh raspberries
75g (3oz) fresh blueberries
4 radishes, thinly sliced
50g (2oz) blue cheese, crumbled

Dressing:
3 tbsp olive oil
2 tbsp lemon juice
2 tsp grated lemon zest
1 tsp sugar substitute
1 tbsp chopped fresh basil
1 tbsp chopped fresh parsley
1 tbsp chopped fresh mint
¼ tsp each sea salt and pepper

1. In a large bowl, toss together the escarole, raspberries, blueberries and radishes.

Dressing: In a bowl, whisk together the olive oil, lemon juice, lemon zest, sugar substitute and seasoning to taste then mix in the herbs.

2. Pour the dressing over the salad and toss gently to coat. Sprinkle with the blue cheese and toss again.

COTTAGE CHEESE AND FRUIT (1 serving)

Perfect for a lunch on the run.

225g (8oz) low-fat cottage cheese
175g (6oz) approx. chopped, fresh fruit or fruit canned in juice, such as peaches, apricots or pears

Place the cottage cheese and fruit in a plastic bowl with a fitted lid and stir to mix. Store in the refrigerator until lunchtime. Enjoy.

VARIATION:
Add a tablespoon of high-fruit, no-added-sugar fruit spread or preserve instead of the chopped fruit.

DINNER

All of the following meal ideas are based on the Gi Diet portion sizes and ratios discussed earlier. Vegetables should take up 50% of your plate – I recommend a mixture. Meat, poultry or fish should take up 25% of your plate and rice, pasta or potatoes should take up the remaining 25%.

STUFFED PEPPERS (4 servings)
Here's a twist on a classic comfort dish.

350g (12oz) lean beef mince
2 cloves garlic, crushed
1 onion, chopped
1 free-range egg, beaten
150g (5oz) pearl barley
2 tbsp tomato purée
½ tsp each sea salt and pepper
4 large peppers (any colour)
1 x 410g (14oz) can good quality tomato pasta sauce

1. In a bowl, mix together the beef, garlic, onion, egg, barley, tomato purée and seasoning.

2. Cut the top off each pepper and remove the seeds and fleshy 'ribs'. Fill each pepper with the beef mixture, pressing in lightly. Discard the tops, seeds and fleshy 'ribs'. Place in a large saucepan to fit snugly and add just enough water to cover the top of peppers. (Don't worry if they turn on their sides during cooking, the filling will stay put.) Bring to a boil then reduce the heat and simmer for 45 minutes, or until barley is tender.

3. Remove peppers from water and place on serving platter. (The peppers can be prepared up to this point, covered and chilled up to 1 day then reheated until piping hot.) Heat pasta sauce and pour over the peppers to serve.

TOMATO AND CHEESE FISH (4 servings)

An easy mid-week dish. Serve it over pasta with a side salad.

4 fillets firm white fish, e.g. hake, or pollack or cod – about 125g (4½oz) each
2 medium tomatoes, chopped
1 sweet onion (such as Vidalia), chopped
1 clove garlic, crushed
1 small red fresh chilli, deseeded and chopped finely
2 tbsp lemon juice
1 tbsp grated lemon zest
2 tsp olive oil
¼ tsp each sea salt and pepper
75g (3oz) reduced-fat cheddar cheese, grated

1. Arrange the fish fillets in a shallow baking dish about 32 x 22cm (13 x 9in).

2. Preheat the oven to 220°C, Gas 7. In a bowl, toss together the tomatoes, onion, garlic, chilli, lemon juice, lemon zest, olive oil and seasoning.

3. Top the fish fillets with the tomato mixture and sprinkle with the cheese. Bake for 15–20 minutes or until fish flakes easily with a fork.

SIDE DISHES

Remember that a quarter of your plate should be filled with a carbohydrate such as pasta, rice or boiled new potatoes. Since overcooking tends to raise the Gi level of food, boil pasta until it is just 'al dente', or still firm when bitten, and take rice off the heat before it starts to clump together. Small new potatoes will only take about ten minutes to boil or steam. Vegetables should be tender-crisp.

Here are some hints for preparing your side vegetables.

To boil vegetables:
In a saucepan of boiling water, cook vegetables until they are just tender.

To steam vegetables:
In a saucepan, boil 3cm (1in) of water. Place a steamer basket filled with the vegetables in the saucepan. Cover and steam for 5–7 minutes or until the vegetables are just tender.

To microwave vegetables:
Place the vegetables in a large plate or bowl. Add 60ml (2fl oz) of water. Cover with cling film and microwave on High for about 5 minutes or until the vegetables are just tender.

It's simple to add some zing to vegetables by drizzling them with lemon juice and adding salt and pepper.

Try these easy-to-prepare green-light suggestions to serve alongside your poultry, fish or meat, for dinner.

• Green beans sprinkled with almonds or mushrooms, rice and salad.
• Basmati rice (you can stir some extra vegetables into the rice during the last minute of cooking). Limit serving size to 50g (2oz) dry weight.
• Pasta, covering a quarter of the plate – about 40g (1½oz) dry weight.
• Boiled new potatoes (2–3 per serving) tossed with herbs and a smidgen of olive oil.
• Mixed vegetables, such as sliced carrots, broccoli or cauliflower florets and halved Brussels sprouts.

Here are two side dishes you might like to try:

MEDITERRANEAN OVEN-ROASTED TOMATOES (4 servings)
These tomatoes are a useful accompaniment to grilled fish or meat. They are also great for lunch paired with some lean ham, cottage cheese and a slice of high-fibre wholegrain bread.

4 large tomatoes
3 anchovy fillets, chopped
2 tbsp olive oil
1 clove garlic, crushed

1 tbsp Dijon mustard
1 tbsp balsamic vinegar
¼ tsp ground black pepper
2 tbsp chopped fresh basil

1. Preheat the oven to 200°C, Gas 6 . Cut the tomatoes in half across the wide middle and place, cut-side up, in a shallow baking dish.

2. In small bowl, beat together the anchovies, olive oil, garlic, mustard, vinegar and pepper. Spoon evenly over tomatoes. Bake for 25–30 minutes or until tomatoes are very soft and wrinkled. Sprinkle basil over the top, cool until warm, not hot, and serve.

OVEN-BAKED COURGETTE COINS (4–6 servings)
A tasty light and healthy starter, snack or side dish.

60g (2¼oz) wholemeal flour
120g (4oz) cornmeal or polenta
2 tbsp finely grated Parmesan cheese
½ tsp each sea salt and pepper
4 medium courgettes, cut into 1cm (½in) rounds
2 egg whites, lightly beaten
A little olive oil, for brushing

1. Preheat the oven to 250°C, Gas 8/9. In a large plastic food bag, shake together the flour, cornmeal, Parmesan and seasoning.

2. Dip the courgette slices first in egg whites then shake in the bag to coat. Brush a baking sheet with some olive oil and arrange the courgettes in a single layer on the sheet. Bake for about 15 minutes, flipping over halfway through until golden brown and crisp.

Poultry

Naturally low in fat, cooked chicken or turkey breast can be used in dozens of ways, combined with a variety of herbs, spices and vegetables to enhance their flavour.

Here's a basic green-light method for cooking poultry.

You'll need:
• Vegetable-oil cooking spray (preferably rapeseed or olive oil)
• 110g (4oz) skinless, boneless chicken breast or turkey breast, whole, sliced or cubed.

Spray oil in a small non-stick frying pan, and then place it over medium-high heat.

Add the chicken or turkey breast and sauté until firm to the touch and no longer pink, about 4 minutes per side for 1 chicken breast or piece of turkey or 5–6 minutes in total for slices or cubes. Set poultry aside.

Here are just two ideas to use cooked chicken:

ITALIAN CHICKEN (2 servings)

225g (8oz) sliced mushrooms
1 medium onion, sliced
1 can (400g/14oz) chopped Italian tomatoes
1 clove garlic, minced
Chopped fresh or dried oregano and basil
225g (8oz) cooked, skinless, boneless, chicken breast or turkey breast

1. Place the mushrooms, onion and tomatoes in a saucepan.

2. Stir in a little water, to prevent the tomatoes from sticking, and heat over medium-low heat until the mushrooms and onion are softened.

3. Add the garlic, oregano and basil, stir to mix, then let simmer for 5 minutes.

4. Add the cooked chicken or turkey and stir to mix. Let simmer until the chicken or turkey is heated through, then serve.

CHICKEN CURRY (2 servings)

Vegetable-oil cooking spray (preferably rapeseed or olive oil)
1 medium onion, sliced
1–2 tsp curry powder, or more to own taste
110g (4oz) sliced carrots
110g (4oz) chopped celery
50g (2oz) uncooked basmati rice
1 medium apple, chopped
25g (1oz) raisins
225g (8oz) cooked, skinless, boneless, chicken breast or turkey breast

1. Spray oil in a non-stick lidded frying pan, then place it over medium heat. Add the onion and curry powder, stir to coat the onion with the curry powder, then sauté for 1 minute.

2. Add the carrots and celery, stir to mix, then sauté for 1 minute.

3. Add the rice, apple, raisins, and 1 cup of water, and stir to mix.

4. Cover the pan and let the curry simmer until all of the liquid is absorbed.

5. Add the cooked chicken or turkey and stir to mix. Keep over heat until the chicken or turkey is heated through, about 2 minutes, then serve.

Fish

Fish is also an excellent source of protein as well as being quick and easy to prepare and cook. Virtually any fish is suitable, but never use commercially breaded or battered versions. Salmon and trout are great favourites in our house. Fish can be pepped up with spice rubs and herbs.

Cooking fish fillets in a microwave oven couldn't be easier. For each person, you'll need one fish fillet (110–150g /4–5oz), sprinkled with 1–2 tsp fresh lemon juice and black pepper to taste. Since the cooking time for fish is critical, the power of microwave ovens varies enormously and more fillets cooked at the same time will take longer to cook, refer to the instructions that came with your microwave for precise cooking times.

VARIATIONS:
• Sprinkle fish with fresh or dried herbs such as dill, parsley, basil and tarragon.
• Cook fish on a bed of leeks and onions. Do not use oil.
• Sprinkle fish with a mixture of wholewheat breadcrumbs and parsley (1 tbsp per fillet) plus 1 tsp melted low-fat non-hydrogenated spread.

Meat

Red meat in general is a yellow-light food, although, for pragmatic reasons, I've included lean cuts of beef and extra-lean minced beef in Phase I. Other red meats such as pork and lamb tend to have a higher fat content.

Serving size is critical. Remember, use the palm of your hand or a pack of playing cards as a guide to your portion size.

For a complete steak-based meal, try the following:

• Grill or barbecue a fully trimmed lean steak (110g/4oz per person).
• Sauté half a sliced onion and 50–75g (2–3oz) mushrooms in a non-stick pan with a little water.
• Microwave, for approximately 3–5 minutes, broccoli, asparagus and Brussels sprouts (approximately 275g/10oz per person) with a little water, seasoned with nutmeg and pepper.
• Boil 50g (2oz) dry basmati rice, or 2–3 boiled new potatoes per person. Season the potatoes with herbs and a touch of olive oil.

BEEF CHILLI (2 servings)

2 tsp olive oil
1 large onion, sliced
2 cloves of garlic, minced
225g (8oz) extra-lean minced beef
2 green peppers, chopped
1 can (410g/14oz) tomatoes
Chilli powder to taste
¼ tsp cayenne (optional)
¼ tsp salt
¼ tsp basil
450ml (16fl oz) water
1 large can (410g/14oz) red kidney beans, rinsed
1 large can (410g/14oz) haricot beans, rinsed

1. Add oil to a deep frying pan or saucepan and sauté onion and garlic until nearly tender.

2. Add minced beef and cook, breaking up with spoon, until browned; drain off any fat.

3. Add green peppers, tomatoes, chilli powder, cayenne (optional), salt, basil and water and bring to the boil. Simmer uncovered until it has reached desired consistency (1–2 hours).

4. Prior to serving, add the red kidney beans and haricot beans. You can garnish this chilli with chopped tomato, fresh parsley, fresh coriander and yoghurt cheese.

VARIATION:
If you're looking for a green-light alternative to sour cream to serve with your chilli, try Yoghurt Cheese (see recipe on page 86). For a vegetarian option, omit the beef from the recipe.

Snacks
Most popular snack foods are disastrous from a sugar and fat standpoint. Commercial biscuits, cakes and chocolate bars should be avoided at all costs. Fortunately, there are equally satisfying alternatives that are both convenient and low-cost. And remember never to leave home without them.

These green-light snacks require no preparation on your part.
1 apple, pear, peach or orange
110g (4oz) low-fat cottage cheese (1% fat or less) with 1 tbsp reduced-sugar jam
175g (6oz) fruit yoghurt with sugar substitute
½ high-protein food bar such as Myoplex/Slim-Fast bars (200 calories; 20–30g carbohydrates; 12–15g protein; 5g fat per bar)

Here are several more delicious snack recipes.

SAVOURY BISCOTTI (Makes about 20. 1 biscotti = 1 serving)

Dunk these savoury treats in soup or serve as a mid-afternoon snack with some raw veggies and cottage cheese. If your sun-dried tomatoes are very dry, soften them in hot water for 5 minutes, drain and squeeze dry.

175g (6oz) wholemeal flour
20g (³⁄₄oz) wheat bran
About 8–10 sun-dried tomatoes, finely chopped
2 tbsp grated Parmesan cheese
1 tsp baking powder
½ tsp bicarbonate of soda
1 tsp dried oregano
1 tsp ground black pepper
2 free-range medium eggs
4 tbsp olive oil

1. Preheat the oven to 180°C, Gas 4. In a large bowl, stir together the flour, wheat bran, sun-dried tomatoes, Parmesan, baking powder, bicarbonate of soda, oregano and pepper.

2. In another bowl, whisk together the eggs, olive oil and 2–3 tbsp cold water then mix into the flour mixture to form a moist but not sticky dough.

3. Divide the dough into 2 equal portions and place on a baking sheet lined with baking parchment. With lightly floured hands, press each portion into a log about 5–6cm (2–2½in) wide, flattening the tops slightly and making sure there are no air pockets.

4. Bake for 20 minutes or until just firm. Remove and cool for 10 minutes.

5. Reduce oven heat to 160°C, Gas 3. Using a serrated knife, cut the logs on a diagonal into 1cm (½in) thick slices. Place back on the baking sheet, leaving a 2.5cm (1in) space between each. Bake until completely dry and crunchy, about 25 minutes, turning once.

CREAMY LEMON SQUARES (Makes 36 squares. 2 squares = 1 serving)

These tiny treats are the ideal mid-afternoon pick-me-up.

Base:
60g (2¼oz) wholemeal flour
20g (¾oz) wheat bran
20g (¾oz) ground almonds
4 tbsp sugar substitute
4 tbsp non-hydrogenated soft-fat spread

Filling:
3 free-range medium eggs, beaten
16 tbsp sugar substitute
125ml (4½fl oz) fresh lemon juice
4 tsp buttermilk
2 tsp lemon zest
2 tsp cornflour
1 tsp baking powder

1. Preheat the oven to 180°C, Gas 4. For the base, mix together in a bowl or food processor the flour, wheat bran, almonds and sugar substitute. Rub in the fat until the mixture is crumbly.

2. Press the mixture evenly into the bottom of a greased non-stick 20cm (8in) square baking pan and bake for 20–25 minutes or until lightly browned. Set aside to cool.

For the filling, whisk together the egg and sugar substitute then stir in lemon juice, buttermilk, lemon zest, cornflour and baking powder. Pour over base and return to the oven for 15–20 minutes or until filling is set.

3. Allow to cool to room temperature, then chill for about 2 hours before cutting into squares.

Storage: Store in an airtight container in the fridge for up to 3 days or freeze for up to 1 month.

BANANA BREAD (Makes 1 loaf/10 to 12 slices. 1 slice = 1 serving)
Try a slice of this quick-bread spread with a teaspoon of light cream cheese.

180g (6oz) wholemeal flour
50g (2oz) ground flaxseed
1 tsp ground cinnamon
2 tsp baking powder
1 tsp bicarbonate of soda
½ tsp sea salt
2 very-ripe (spotty) bananas, mashed
12 tbsp sugar substitute
185 ml (6½fl oz) buttermilk
2 free-range eggs
1 tsp vanilla extract

1. Preheat the oven to 180°C, Gas 4. Grease a 1kg (2¼lb) non-stick loaf tin. In a bowl, mix together the flour, flaxseed, cinnamon, baking powder, bicarbonate of soda and salt.

2. In another bowl, mix together bananas, sugar substitute, buttermilk, eggs and vanilla. Pour into flour mixture and stir until just moistened.

3. Pour the batter into the prepared loaf tin. Bake for 45–50 minutes or until a thin metal skewer inserted in the centre comes out clean. Cool on a wire rack and serve in slices.

Wrap in cling film or foil and store at room temperature for up to 3 days or wrap in freezer cling film and heavy-duty foil and freeze for up to 1 month.

Desserts

The good news is that dessert should be part of your diet – but not the guilt-inducing kind loaded with sugar and fats. Fortunately, there is a broad range of low-Gi, low-calorie alternatives that taste good and are good for you. Virtually any fruit qualifies (though hold off on the raisins and bananas) and there are numerous low-fat dairy products such as yoghurt and ice cream that are sweetened with sweetener rather than sugar. You'll also find some delicious recipes in this book.

7 Phase I – the 7-day Plan

Here are some ideas for a 7-day Phase I menu plan, to show you just some of the delicious meals and snacks that you can prepare to eat the Gi way.

Where you see an asterisk (*) in the text, this means you'll find the recipe in this book.

Each day, include a mid-morning and a mid-afternoon snack. For the purposes of this plan, I'm making your third 'snack' your evening dessert.

DAY 1

Breakfast:
* Porridge topped with a small carton of 'diet' raspberry yoghurt and 2 tbsp slivered almonds
A whole orange (not just the juice)
1 cup decaffeinated coffee or tea

Morning snack:
Light cottage cheese with fruit

Lunch:
Either * Haricot Bean Soup and green salad, or

* Crab salad in Tomato Shells with ½ wholemeal pitta bread

Afternoon snack:
*Savoury Biscotti

Dinner:
* Beef Cutlets in Mushroom Gravy, with boiled new potatoes and green beans

Evening snack:
* Berry Crumble

DAY 2

Breakfast:
* Homemade Breakfast Muesli.
2 slices lean back bacon
1 slice 100% stone-ground wholemeal toast spread with 2 teaspoon low-fat unsaturated spread
1 cup decaffeinated coffee or tea

Morning snack:
*A slice of Banana Bread

Lunch:
Either * Mushroom Barley and Beef Soup and green salad, or
* Barbecue-Chicken Salad

1 orange

Afternoon snack:
Carrots, cucumber, sliced peppers with hummus

Dinner:
* Grilled Pesto Salmon with Asparagus and new potatoes, or rice and salad

Evening snack:
* Poached Pears with Sweetened Yoghurt Cheese

DAY 3

Breakfast:
* 4 Buttermilk Pancakes, topped with 100g red berries
A small carton of 'diet' strawberry yoghurt.
1 cup decaffeinated coffee or tea

Morning snack:
Fruit yoghurt and fresh berries

Lunch:
* Tangy Red-and-Green Coleslaw
Either * Smoked-Trout Pâté, with wholewheat crackers or pitta bread

or an
* Open-Faced Sandwich

Afternoon snack:
A small wholemeal scone

Dinner:
* White Chicken Chilli, with rice and green salad.

Evening snack:
* Apple-Sauce Cookies

DAY 4

Breakfast:
* Crunchy Baked French Toast
1 orange
1 cup decaffeinated coffee or tea

Morning snack:
Half a high-protein nutrition bar

Lunch:
• Minestrone Soup and salad

Afternoon snack:
Apple and almonds

Dinner:
* Vegetarian Shepherd's Pie, with carrots, green vegetables and salad

Evening snack:
* Peach Meringue

DAY 5

Breakfast:
* Morning Glory Poached Fruit
1 slice 100% stone-ground wholemeal toast spread with 2 teaspoons low-fat unsaturated spread and 1 tablespoon reduced-sugar jam
1 cup decaffeinated coffee or tea

Morning snack:
* Creamy Lemon Squares

Lunch:
Either * Ham and Lentil Soup and

salad or
* Fennel Waldorf Salad
½ wholemeal pitta bread

Afternoon snack:
Fruit yoghurt and almonds

Dinner:
* Thai-Style Tofu and Broccoli, with rice or wholewheat pasta and salad

Evening snack:
* Almond Crusted Pears or a * Chocolate Drop Cookie

DAY 6

Breakfast:
* Wheat Grain Breakfast
1 slice 100% stone-ground whole-meal toast spread with 2 teaspoons low-fat unsaturated spread and 1 tablespoon reduced-sugar jam.
1 orange
1 cup decaffeinated coffee or tea

Morning snack:
*Chocolate Drop Cookie

Lunch:
Either * Smoky Black Bean Soup and salad, or
* Open-Faced Reuben Sandwich with salad

Afternoon snack:
A bowl of fresh fruit salad

Dinner:
* Chilled Spinach and Watercress Soup
* Quick Fish (see recipe on page 71) Steaks with Tomato-Chickpea Relish, new potatoes and green beans

Evening snack:
* Grilled Fruit Kebabs with Lemon-Yoghurt Sauce

DAY 7

Breakfast:
* Homey Oatmeal topped with a chopped pear and a handful of red berries
1 orange
1 cup decaffeinated coffee or tea

Morning snack:
*Apple-Sauce Cookie

Lunch:
Either * Tuscan White-Bean Soup and salad, or
* Open-Faced Chicken or Turkey Sandwich

Pepper, cucumber and celery sticks with * Roasted Red-Pepper Hummus

Afternoon snack:
2 mini light Babybel cheeses and a pear

Dinner:
* Chicken Tagine, with basmati rice and salad

Evening snack:
* Pecan Brownie, with fresh peach and 'diet' peach yoghurt

7 DAY PLAN – RECIPES

DAY 1

PORRIDGE (1 serving)
50g (2oz) large-flake oats
225ml (8fl oz) water or skimmed milk
150–175g (5–6oz) 'diet' fruit yoghurt
2 tbsp sliced almonds
Fresh fruit

Cover oats with water or milk. Microwave on medium setting for 3 minutes. Mix in yoghurt, almonds and fresh fruit.

Top the meal off with an orange and a glass of skimmed milk and you have a delicious breakfast that will stay with you all morning.

HARICOT BEAN SOUP (4 servings)
This recipe comes from Beth F., who went on the Gi Diet after hearing about it on a local radio show. She and her husband are both enjoying the new way of eating and like having this thick and nourishing soup for lunch.

3 litres (5 pints) water
320g (11oz) dried haricot beans
2 carrots, chopped
1 large onion, chopped
1 celery stalk, chopped
1 bay leaf
1 tsp salt
1 pinch pepper
Tabasco sauce (optional)

1. Into a large stockpot, pour 2 litres (3½ pints) of the water, add the haricot beans and bring to the boil. Reduce the heat and simmer for about 1 hour or until the beans are almost tender.

2. Add the remaining water, carrots, onion, celery stalk and bay leaf and cook for about 1 hour or until the vegetables and beans are tender. Remove the bay leaf. Add the salt and pepper. Serve with Tabasco, if desired.

CRAB SALAD IN TOMATO SHELLS (4 servings)

Beefsteak tomatoes are ideal for this dish because their large size will accommodate the filling and because their pulp and seeds are easy to scoop out. Try using shrimps or small prawns, tuna or salmon instead of the crab.

2 packages (each 200g/7oz) frozen crab, thawed
4 large beefsteak tomatoes
60ml (2fl oz) low-fat mayonnaise
2 tbsp light sour cream
½ tsp finely grated lemon rind
1 tbsp lemon juice
2 tsp chopped fresh tarragon or ½ tsp dried
1 pinch each salt and pepper
225g (8oz) coarsely chopped cooked chickpeas
½ red pepper, diced
25g (1oz) finely diced celery
10g (½oz) chopped fresh flat-leaf parsley
2 tbsp chopped fresh chives
2 tbsp shredded carrot

1. Place the crab in a fine mesh sieve and press out any liquid. Remove any cartilage if necessary and set aside.

2. Cut the top quarter off the tomatoes. Using a small spoon, scoop out the seeds and pulp. Place the tomatoes cut-side down on a paper-towel-lined plate.

3. Meanwhile, in a large bowl, whisk together the mayonnaise, sour cream, lemon rind and juice, tarragon, salt and pepper. Add the chickpeas, red pepper, celery, parsley, chives and carrot. Then add the crab and stir to combine. Divide the crab mixture among the tomatoes.

VARIATIONS:
Herb option: Substitute an additional 3 tbsp chopped flat-leaf parsley for the chives and tarragon.

Seafood option: Substitute 350g (12oz) crabsticks, chopped finely, or prawns, or 2 cans (110g/4oz each) tuna or salmon, for the crabmeat.

Crab melts: Omit the tomatoes. Top 4 slices of stone-ground wholemeal bread with the crab mixture and sprinkle with 40g (1½oz) of shredded light-style Swiss cheese. Place them under the grill until melted. This makes a great lunch for 4 people.

BEEF CUTLETS IN MUSHROOM GRAVY (4 servings)

1 free-range egg
4 savoury wheat crackers, e.g.
Krackawheat, crushed finely
½ carrot, grated
12 pitted black or green olives,
chopped
2 cloves garlic, crushed
1 tsp Worcestershire sauce

½ tsp ground black pepper
¼ tsp sea salt
350g (12oz) lean minced beef
2 tsp olive oil
1 large onion, sliced
250g (9oz) mushrooms, sliced
500ml (18fl oz) beef stock
1 tbsp tomato purée

1. In a large bowl, whisk the egg then mix in the crackers, carrot, olives, garlic, Worcestershire sauce, black pepper and salt. Then mix in the beef with your hands. Form the meat mixture into 4 oval patties, each about 2 cm (¾in) thick. Heat a greased grill pan or non-stick frying pan and fry the patties for about 3–4 minutes per side until browned.

2. Meanwhile, heat oil in a large non-stick frying pan over medium-high heat and cook the onions and mushrooms until softened and turning golden, about 8 minutes. Stir in the beef stock and tomato purée. Bring to the boil, add the beef patties, cover and simmer for 10 minutes until firm when pressed. Serve with new potatoes and green beans.

BERRY CRUMBLE (6 servings)

700g (1½lb) fresh or frozen berries
– raspberries, blackberries, blueberries and sliced strawberries
1 large apple, cored and chopped
2 tbsp wholemeal flour
2 tbsp sugar substitute
½ tsp cinnamon

Topping:
110g (4oz) large-flake oats
50g (2oz) chopped pecans or
walnuts
4 tbsp sugar substitute
50g (2oz) non-hydrogenated
spread, melted
1 tsp cinnamon

1. In a 20cm (8in) square baking dish, combine the berries and apple. In a bowl, combine the flour, sugar substitute and cinnamon. Sprinkle this over the fruit and toss gently.

2. Topping: In a bowl, combine the oats, pecans, sugar substitute, spread and cinnamon. Sprinkle this over the fruit mixture. Bake in a 180°C, Gas 4, oven for about 30 minutes or until the fruit is tender and the top is golden.

Microwave option: Prepare as above and microwave on High for about 6 minutes or until fruit is tender. The top won't get golden or crisp.

DAY 2

HOMEMADE BREAKFAST MUESLI (450g/ 1lb)

My friend Lesleigh introduced me to this delicious and healthy start to the day. Be sure to prepare it the night before so that it's ready to enjoy in the morning. Combine 75g (3oz) of the muesli with 60ml (2fl oz) of skimmed milk or water, and cover and refrigerate overnight. Then, in the morning, combine the mixture with 1 carton (175g) of 'diet' yoghurt and enjoy it cold, or pop it in the microwave for a hot breakfast.

200g (7oz) large-flake oats
75g (3oz) oat bran
75g (3oz) sliced almonds
50g (2oz) unsalted sunflower seeds
2 tbsp wheat germ
¼ tsp cinnamon

In a large, resealable plastic bag, combine the oats, oat bran, almonds, sunflower seeds, wheat germ and cinnamon. Using a rolling pin, crush the mixture into coarse crumbs. Shake the bag to combine the mixture.

Storage: Keep in a resealable bag or airtight container at room temperature for up to 1 month.

MUSHROOM, BARLEY AND BEEF SOUP (4–6 servings)
A thick, hearty stew-like soup will warm up anyone on a cold winter's night. This is real comfort food for the soul and the belly.

1 tbsp rapeseed oil
225g (8oz) extra-lean minced beef
1 onion, chopped
2 cloves garlic, crushed
450g (1lb) mushrooms, sliced
1 each carrot and celery stalk, chopped
1 tbsp chopped fresh thyme leaves or 1 tsp dried thyme
2 tbsp tomato paste
1 tbsp balsamic vinegar
¼ tsp each salt and pepper
900ml (1½ pints) beef stock (low-fat, low-sodium)
600ml (1¼ pints) water
110g (4oz) barley
1 bay leaf
1 can (410g) black beans, drained and rinsed

1. In a large stockpot, heat the oil over a medium-high heat and cook the beef until it is no longer pink. Reduce the heat to medium and add the onion and garlic; cook, stirring, for 5 minutes. Add the mushrooms, carrot, celery and thyme and cook for about 15 minutes or until all the liquid has evaporated from the mushrooms.

2. Add the tomato paste, balsamic vinegar, salt and pepper; stir to coat the vegetables.

3. Add the stock, water, barley and bay leaf; bring to the boil. Reduce the heat, cover and simmer for about 45 minutes or until the barley is tender. Add the beans and heat through. Remove the bay leaf.

VARIATIONS:
Chicken option: You can use minced chicken or turkey instead of the beef and use chicken stock instead of beef stock.

Note: Mushrooms come in all shapes and sizes. The best for this soup are white or brown button mushrooms, shiitakes, oyster or even Portobellos.

BARBECUE-CHICKEN SALAD (4 servings)

You can add the chicken to this salad hot off the grill, or barbecue it ahead of time and use it cold. For a packed lunch, stuff it into half a whole-wheat pitta.

2 tbsp soy sauce
2 tbsp rapeseed oil
2 tbsp chopped fresh coriander
1 tbsp crushed fresh ginger
2 cloves garlic, crushed
¼ tsp Asian chilli paste or red-pepper flakes
4 boneless skinless chicken breasts
2 each red and yellow peppers
175g (6oz) mixed salad leaves
3 tbsp rice vinegar
¼ tsp salt

1. In a large bowl, whisk together the soy sauce, 1 tbsp of the oil, the coriander, ginger, garlic and chilli paste or red-pepper flakes. Add the chicken breasts and toss everything to coat it well. Cover and refrigerate for at least 30 minutes or up to 1 day.

2. Meanwhile, cut the peppers into quarters. Place them in a greased grill pan under a medium-high heat. Grill them for about 15 minutes, turning once, or until they start to blacken. Remove them to a plate. Place the chicken breasts in a greased grill pan under a medium-high heat and grill them for about 12 minutes, turning once, or until no longer pink inside. Place them on a plate.

3. Chop the grilled peppers and chicken into bite-size pieces. In a large bowl, toss the chicken and peppers with the mixed salad leaves, the remaining oil and the rice vinegar and salt.

VARIATIONS:
Roasting option: You can roast the peppers and chicken instead of grilling them. Place the vegetables on a parchment-paper–lined baking tray and roast them in a 225°C, Gas 7, pre-heated oven for about 15 minutes. Add the chicken breasts and roast for another 12 minutes or until the chicken is no longer pink inside and the peppers are blackened.

Storage: This salad will last up to 1 day in the refrigerator.

GRILLED PESTO SALMON WITH ASPARAGUS (4 servings)

60ml (2fl oz) light mayonnaise
2 tbsp chopped fresh flat-leaf
parsley
1 tbsp pesto
1 pinch each salt and pepper
4 boneless salmon fillets, skin on,
each 120g (4oz)
450g (1lb) asparagus spears
2 tsp extra-virgin olive oil
¼ tsp pepper
2 tbsp lemon juice
¼ tsp salt

1. In a small bowl, whisk together the mayonnaise, parsley, pesto and salt and pepper. Spread it evenly over the top of the salmon.

2. Snap off the tough ends of asparagus and discard. Toss the spears with oil and pepper.

3. Place the fillets and asparagus in a greased grill pan under a medium-high heat. Grill for about 10 minutes or until the fish is firm to the touch and the asparagus is tender-crisp. Drizzle the asparagus with lemon juice and sprinkle with salt.

VARIATION:
Fish options: This pesto mixture is delicious on halibut, tuna or trout.

Helpful hint: Leaving the skin on the fillets helps the fish stay moist and keeps it from falling apart.

POACHED PEARS (2 servings)
Serve these pears with a dollop of Yoghurt Cheese (see recipe on page 86) or low-fat, no-added-sugar ice cream.

420ml (¾ pint) pear juice
4 black peppercorns
2 whole cloves
1 cinnamon stick
2 pears, cored and quartered

1. In a saucepan, bring the pear juice, peppercorns, cloves and cinnamon stick to the boil. Reduce the heat to simmer and add the pears.

2. Simmer for about 10 minutes or until the pears are tender when pierced with a knife. Place them in a bowl.

3. Boil the juice mixture again for 3 minutes. Strain over the pears.

YOGHURT CHEESE (Makes 350g/ 12oz)

This can be used as a tasty spread for wholemeal toast in the morning, as a dip, or as a topping for a dessert. Yoghurt cheese is also a great substitute for sour cream in most recipes.

1 large carton (750g) plain low-fat yoghurt

Empty the yoghurt into a sieve lined with cheesecloth or a clean tea towel. Place it over a large bowl. Cover it all with cling film and refrigerate for at least 4 hours or overnight. Discard any liquid and place the yoghurt cheese in an airtight container.

VARIATIONS:
Sweet Yoghurt Cheese: You can sweeten your yoghurt cheese by adding some sugar substitute to taste.

Lemony Yoghurt Cheese: Add 1 tsp grated lemon rind and 2 tsp lemon juice along with the sugar substitute to taste.

Quick Yoghurt Cheese Dip: Simply add 2 spring onions, chopped; 1 small clove garlic, crushed; 1 tbsp lemon juice; and 1 tbsp chopped fresh oregano (or 1 tsp dried) to the yoghurt cheese.

Helpful hint: Keep the container the yoghurt came in and write down the best-before date – that's how long your yoghurt cheese is good for.

DAY 3

BUTTERMILK PANCAKES (about 16 pancakes, enough for 4–6 servings)
This recipe comes from Michelle R. Though buttermilk may sound as though it's rich and indulgent, it's actually low in fat and adds a wonderful tang to these pancakes.

225g (8oz) wholemeal flour
1 tsp baking powder
2 tsp sugar substitute
420ml (¾ pint) buttermilk
2 omega-3 eggs
2 tbsp rapeseed oil
½ tsp vanilla essence

1. In a large bowl, combine the flour, baking powder and sugar substitute. In another bowl, whisk together the buttermilk, eggs, oil and vanilla essence. Pour the buttermilk mixture over the flour mixture and whisk together until smooth.

2. Heat a large non-stick frying pan over a medium heat. Ladle the batter into the pan. Cook it for about 2 minutes or until bubbles appear on top of the pancake. Using a spatula, flip the pancake and cook for another minute or until golden. Repeat with the remaining batter.

TANGY RED-AND-GREEN COLESLAW (4–6 servings)
Using a vinaigrette in coleslaw makes it low fat and really tangy! This salad keeps well in the refrigerator.

325g (11oz) finely shredded green cabbage
160g (5½oz) finely shredded red cabbage
2 carrots, shredded
60g (2½oz) thinly sliced celery
10g (½oz) chopped flat-leaf parsley

110ml (4fl oz) cider vinegar
2 tbsp rapeseed oil
2 tsp sugar substitute
1 tsp celery seeds
½ tsp salt
1 pinch pepper

1. In a large bowl, toss together the green and red cabbage, carrots, celery and parsley.

2. In a small bowl, whisk together the vinegar, oil, sugar substitute, celery seeds, salt and pepper. Pour it over the cabbage mixture and toss to coat.

Storage: Cover and refrigerate for up to 2 days.

VARIATIONS:
Creamy coleslaw dressing option: Whisk together 60ml (2fl oz) each plain yoghurt and light mayonnaise, 2 tbsp cider vinegar, 1 tbsp Dijon mustard, 2 tsp sugar substitute, 1/2 tsp celery seed and 1/4 tsp salt.

OPEN-FACED LUNCH SANDWICHES (2 servings)
These delicious sandwiches are chock full of protein and vegetables. For a change, substitute the bread with pitta halves.

4 slices stone-ground wholemeal bread
1/2 ripe avocado, peeled and stoned
105g (4oz) cooked chickpeas, chopped
50g (2oz) Light Boursin or Laughing Cow Light cheese
2 tbsp freshly chopped basil or flat-leaf parsley
1/4 tsp each salt and freshly ground black pepper
4 slices lean ham or turkey (optional)
1/2 cucumber, chopped
1 plum tomato, chopped
25g (1oz) grated carrot
1 tbsp red-wine vinegar
1/4 tsp dried oregano

1. Toast the bread slices in the toaster or under the grill.

2. In a bowl, using a fork, mash the avocado until almost smooth. Add the chickpeas, cheese, parsley and half of the salt and pepper. Divide and spread over the bread. Top with ham or turkey, if desired.

3. In a bowl, combine the cucumber, tomato, carrot, red-wine vinegar, oregano and remaining salt and pepper. Divide evenly on the bread.

VARIATION:
Tuna option: Omit the ham (if using) and add 1 can (120g) tuna to the cucumber mixture to serve on bread or in pitta.

SMOKED-TROUT PÂTÉ (4–6 servings)

Spread this on open-faced sandwiches, whole-wheat crackers or lightly toasted pitta breads.

350g (12oz) smoked-trout fillets, broken into chunks
50g (2oz) light cream cheese, softened
1 shallot, finely chopped
2 tbsp horseradish relish
2 tbsp fresh lemon juice
½ tsp ground black pepper

In a food processor, whiz the trout with the cream cheese, shallot, horse-radish, lemon juice and pepper until smooth. Chill for up to 3 days.

WHITE CHICKEN CHILLI (4–6 servings)

4 skinless, boneless chicken breasts, about 125g (4½oz) each
2 tsp olive oil
About 200g (7oz) shredded cabbage
3 cloves garlic, crushed
2 onions, chopped
1 carrot, chopped
1 jalapeno pepper or large fresh green chilli (optional), seeded and chopped finely
600ml (1pint) chicken stock
1 x 410g can cannellini beans, drained
2 tsp ground cumin
1 tsp chilli powder
1 tsp dried oregano
¼ tsp sea salt

Toppings (optional):
Good quality pasta sauce
Some chopped fresh coriander
Low-fat natural yoghurt or 0%-fat fromage frais

1. Cut the chicken into bite-size cubes. In a deep frying pan, heat the olive oil over a medium-high heat. Stir-fry the cabbage, garlic, onions, carrot and jalapeno pepper or chilli, if using, for about 10 minutes or until softened. Push the vegetables to the side of pan; add chicken and cook for about 3 minutes until lightly browned.

2. Stir in the stock, beans, cumin, chilli powder, oregano and salt. Cook for 15–20 minutes or until chicken is cooked through.

3. Serve over boiled rice with one or more of the optional toppings.

APPLE-SAUCE COOKIES (about 18 cookies)

These cookies combine all the flavours of a traditional apple pie and have a texture similar to that of a soft granola bar. A great snack!

100g (3 2/3 oz) large-flake oatmeal
90g (3oz) wholemeal flour
1 tsp cinnamon
½ tsp baking powder
1 pinch each nutmeg and salt
240ml (8fl oz) unsweetened apple sauce/purée
6 tbsp sugar substitute
2 omega-3 eggs
2 tsp vanilla essence
1 apple, cored and finely diced

1. In a large bowl, combine the oatmeal, flour, cinnamon, baking powder, nutmeg and salt. In another bowl, whisk together the apple sauce, sugar substitute, eggs and vanilla essence. Pour this over the oatmeal mixture and stir to combine. Add the apple and stir to distribute evenly.

2. Drop heaped tablespoonfuls of the mixture on to a greaseproof-paper-lined baking tray. Bake in a 140°C, Gas 1, oven for about 25 minutes or until firm and lightly golden. Let them cool completely.

Storage: Keep in an airtight container for up to 3 days or freeze for up to 2 weeks.

DAY 4

CRUNCHY BAKED FRENCH TOAST (6 servings)

This crispy, nutty coating takes simple French toast (Eggy toast) to the next level.

25g (1oz) ground almonds
25g (1oz) ground flaxseed
30g (1¼oz) porridge oats
2 tbsp sugar substitute
1 tsp ground cinnamon

4 free-range eggs, beaten
250ml (9fl oz) skimmed milk
1 tsp vanilla extract
6 slices wholemeal bread

1. Preheat the oven to 200°C, Gas 6. Mix together almonds, flaxseed, oats, sugar substitute and cinnamon and tip on to a dinner plate.

2. In shallow medium bowl, whisk together the eggs, milk and vanilla.

3. Dip the bread slices, two at a time, into the egg mixture, turning to coat well then let bread sit in the mixture for 2 minutes. Remove the slices, one at a time, from the mixture and place down on the nut mixture, pressing lightly until nicely coated. Turn the bread over and repeat on the other side then place on a lightly greased baking sheet.

4. Bake for up to 20 minutes, turning halfway through, or until the coating is crisp. Serve with fruit or berries and yoghurt.

MINESTRONE SOUP (6 servings)

This soup is one of my favourites because it contains both pasta and spinach. Serve it with a sprinkling of grated Parmesan for extra flavour and a few more red-pepper flakes to get your blood pumping.

2 tsp rapeseed oil
3 slices back bacon, chopped
1 onion, chopped
4 cloves garlic, crushed
2 carrots, chopped
1 celery stalk, chopped
1 tbsp dried oregano
½ tsp red-pepper flakes
½ tsp each salt and pepper
1 can (410g/14oz) plum tomatoes
1.5 litres (3½ pints) chicken stock

(low-fat, low-sodium)
1 bag (275g/10oz) baby spinach
1 can (410g/14oz) each red kidney beans and chickpeas, drained and rinsed
110g (4oz) ditali or tubetti pasta
10g (½oz) chopped fresh flat-leaf parsley
2 tbsp chopped fresh basil (optional)

1. In a large stockpot, heat the oil over a medium-high heat and cook the back bacon for 2 minutes. Reduce the heat to medium and add the onion, garlic, carrots, celery, oregano, red-pepper flakes, salt and pepper. Cook for about 10 minutes or until softened and just about golden.

2. Add the tomatoes and crush them using a potato masher in the pot. Pour in the chicken stock; bring to the boil. Reduce the heat to a simmer and add the spinach, red kidney beans, chickpeas and pasta. Simmer for about 20 minutes or until the pasta is tender. Stir in the parsley and basil (if desired).

VARIATIONS:
Vegetarian option: Omit the back bacon and use vegetable stock for the chicken stock.

VEGETARIAN SHEPHERD'S PIE (4 servings)
The shepherd ate quite a bit of vegetables and grains, so why not create a favourite meat-filled dish without the meat? Here the base uses bulgur and beans to create a rich and protein-high bottom of our pie. Bulgur is also sold as cracked wheat.

1 tsp rapeseed oil
1 small onion, finely chopped
2 cloves garlic, crushed
110g (4oz) bulgur wheat
1 tsp dried oregano
½ tsp dried basil
400ml (13fl oz) vegetarian simulated 'chicken' stock
200g (7oz) canned tomatoes in juice
2 new red potatoes
1 can (410g/14oz) chickpeas, drained and rinsed
100g (4oz) frozen peas
½ tsp each salt and pepper
2 tbsp chopped flat-leaf parsley

1. In a non-stick frying pan, heat the oil over a medium heat and cook the onion, garlic, bulgur, oregano and basil for about 5 minutes or until the onion is softened and the bulgur is toasted. Add the stock and tomatoes, breaking up the tomatoes with the back of a spoon; bring to the boil and reduce the heat to a simmer. Cover and cook for about 10 minutes or until the bulgur is tender but firm.

2. Meanwhile, pierce the potatoes all over with a fork. Place the potatoes in a small bowl with 60ml (2fl oz) of water and microwave on High for 5 minutes. Allow to cool.

3. Add the chickpeas, peas and half each of the salt and pepper to the bulgur mixture; stir to combine and scrape into an 8in casserole dish, smoothing the top.

4. Thinly slice the potatoes and layer, overlapping slightly, on top of the bulgur mixture. Sprinkle with the remaining salt and pepper and the parsley.

5. Bake in a 200°C, Gas 6, oven for about 20 minutes or until the mixture is bubbly. Let this cool slightly before serving.

VARIATIONS:
Boiled-potato option: In a saucepan, boil the potatoes for about 10 minutes or until tender but firm.

Helpful hint: This dish tastes delicious with the bulgur part on its own, if you don't want to put the potatoes on top. Enjoy!

PEACH MERINGUE (6 servings)
This is an uncomplicated dessert to prepare. To make individual servings, divide the peach mixture and meringue among 6 ovenproof ramekins.

2 x 410g (14oz) cans sliced peaches in juice, drained
1 tbsp sugar substitute, optional
½ tsp ground cinnamon
3 free-range egg whites
¼ tsp cream of tartar
8 tbsp sugar substitute

1. Preheat the oven to 150°C, Gas 2. In a large bowl, mix together the peaches, sugar substitute (if liked) and cinnamon. Spoon into a pie plate or shallow baking dish.

2. In another large bowl, beat the egg whites with the cream of tartar until soft peaks form then gradually beat in the sugar substitute until stiff peaks form.

3. Spread the meringue over the fruit, covering completely. Bake for 30–35 minutes or until golden, turning the dish if the meringue browns too quickly. Serve immediately.

DAY 5

MORNING GLORY POACHED FRUIT (4 servings)

If you don't have time to eat breakfast at home, make this fruit dish the night before, or a few days before, and take it with you. It also makes a wonderful mid-morning or mid-afternoon snack.

Cinnamon Syrup:
450ml (¾ pint) water
2 cinnamon sticks, broken in half
4 slices fresh ginger
3 tbsp sugar substitute

Fruit:
2 apples, cored and coarsely chopped
2 pears, cored and coarsely chopped
1 grapefruit
1 orange
450g (1lb) low-fat cottage cheese or Yoghurt Cheese

1. Cinnamon Syrup: In a small saucepan, bring the water, cinnamon sticks, ginger and sugar substitute to the boil. Reduce the heat to simmer and add the apples and pears. Cook the fruit for about 5 minutes or until just tender. Remove the fruit with a slotted spoon to a large bowl, reserving the syrup. Let it cool.

2. Meanwhile, using a serrated knife, cut both ends off the grapefruit then, starting at one end, peel off the skin and white pith, leaving the fruit intact. Repeat with the orange. Using the same knife, cut the segments between the membranes of the grapefruit and orange and add, along with juices, to the bowl containing the apples and pears. Serve with cottage cheese or Yoghurt Cheese and drizzle with some of the Cinnamon Syrup, if desired.

Storage: You can make this mixture up to 3 days ahead. Store it in an airtight container in the refrigerator.

HAM AND LENTIL SOUP (4 servings)

Tinned lentils make this soup quick and easy to prepare, so keep some on hand in the pantry. If you want to make this soup even more green-light, use dried lentils.

1 tbsp rapeseed oil
1 onion, chopped
50g (2oz) diced celery
2 cloves garlic, crushed
1.5 litres (3½ pints) chicken stock (low-fat, low-sodium)
2 cans (2 x 410g) lentils, drained and rinsed
180g (6oz) Black Forest ham, diced
1 red pepper, diced
2 tomatoes, seeded and diced
2 tbsp chopped fresh flat-leaf parsley

In a large stockpot, heat the oil over a medium heat and cook the onion, celery and garlic for about 5 minutes or until softened. Add the stock, lentils, ham and red pepper; bring to the boil. Reduce the heat and add the tomatoes. Cover and simmer for 20 minutes. Stir in the parsley.

VARIATIONS:
Dried lentil option: Use 200g (7oz) dried green or brown lentils. Add with the stock, and cover and simmer for about 30 minutes or until tender.

THAI-STYLE TOFU AND BROCCOLI (4 servings)

Serve hot or cold over rice or whole-wheat pasta.

350ml (12fl oz) hot vegetable stock
1 stalk lemongrass, finely chopped
1 tbsp rapeseed oil
500g (1lb 2oz) firm tofu, cubed
3 cloves garlic, crushed
1 small hot red chilli pepper, seeded and finely chopped
1 tsp toasted sesame oil
1 head broccoli, cut into florets, stems peeled and chopped
1 red pepper, cored and cut into thin strips
6 tbsp chopped fresh coriander
1 tbsp fresh lime juice
3 spring onions, chopped
2 tbsp soy sauce

1. In a small bowl, pour the stock over the lemongrass and set aside.

2. In wok or large non-stick frying pan, heat the oil over medium-high heat. Add the tofu, garlic, chilli and sesame oil. Stir-fry for 3 minutes or until tofu is starting to turn golden.

3. Add the broccoli, red pepper and lemongrass mixture. Reduce the heat to medium, cover and cook for 5 minutes.

4. Stir in the coriander, lime juice, spring onions and soy sauce then cover and cook for another 2 minutes or until broccoli is just tender.

ALMOND CRUSTED PEARS (4 servings)

This dessert is a great finish to an entertaining meal. The almonds form a crunchy crust on the outside but the pears are tender crisp beneath their coating. Serve some of the juice from the pan alongside the pears.

Pears:
90g (3½oz) flaked almonds
2 tbsp wheat germ
4 tbsp sugar substitute
1 omega-3 egg, beaten
4 ripe Williams or Bosc pears, cored
125ml (4fl oz) pear nectar or juice

Yoghurt Cheese:
250g (9oz) plain low-fat yoghurt
2 tbsp sugar substitute
½ tsp grated orange rind (optional)

1. Make the Yoghurt Cheese (see page 86) using 250g (9oz) plain low-fat yoghurt and 2 tbsp sugar substitute. Flavour the cheese with ½ tsp grated orange rind if desired. Refrigerate.

2. Using your hands, crush the almonds slightly and place in a shallow dish. Add the wheat germ and sugar substitute.

3. Fill the pears with some of the almond mixture. Brush each pear with some of the egg and then roll and press into the remaining almond mixture. Place in a 20cm (8in) square baking dish, standing upright. Pour the pear juice into the bottom of the dish and sprinkle the remaining almond mixture into the pan. Cover lightly with foil and bake in a 200°C, Gas 6, oven for about 30 minutes or until a knife inserts into a pear easily. Remove the foil and bake for another 10 minutes or until golden and the juices have thickened. Let cool slightly. Serve with the Yoghurt Cheese.

CHOCOLATE DROP COOKIES (about 24 cookies)

These are moist cakelets, which, like cookies, are great to eat warm and dunk into a glass of milk for snack time. Made with beans, there is fibre in them that kids won't even know they're getting. Sometimes it pays to be sneaky.

90g (3½oz) non-hydrogenated spread
90g (3½oz) wholemeal flour
8 tbsp sugar substitute
125ml (4fl oz) bean purée (see instructions below)
40g (1½oz) unsweetened cocoa powder
60ml (2fl oz) skimmed milk
1 omega-3 egg
2 tsp vanilla
½ tsp baking powder

1. In a bowl, using an electric beater, beat the spread, flour, sugar substitute, bean purée, cocoa powder, skimmed milk, egg, vanilla and baking powder until combined.

2. Drop tablespoonfuls of the mixture on to a greaseproof-paper-lined baking sheet. Bake in a 190°C, Gas 5, oven for about 10 minutes or until firm to the touch. Let cool.

Storage: Keep in a resealable plastic bag or airtight container for about 3 days at room temperature or in the freezer for up to 3 weeks.

Bean purée: In a food processor, purée 275ml (½ pint) cooked cannellini beans with 2 tbsp wheat bran and 60ml (2fl oz) skimmed milk. Makes enough bean purée for 2 batches of Chocolate Drop Cookies. You can bake a batch now and freeze the remaining bean purée for up to 2 weeks.

DAY 6

WHEAT-GRAIN BREAKFAST (about 3 servings)
This recipe comes from Gi Dieter Gwyneth, who has been making it for many years – especially during canoe trips. You can buy wheat grain, also known as wheat berries, or soft or hard wheat kernels, at health- or bulk-food stores. Letting them sit overnight allows them to crack open, producing a delicate kernel of wheat.

225g (8oz) wheat grain
1 litre (1¾ pints) water
Skimmed milk
Sugar substitute
Slivered almonds
Fresh fruit (such as berries or peaches)

1. Place the wheat grain and water in a saucepan and bring to the boil. Reduce the heat and simmer for 20 minutes.

2. Pour the wheat grain and water mixture into a large vacuum flask, or heatproof airtight container, and seal tightly. Let it stand overnight.

3. Drain any water from the wheat grain. Serve about 90g (3½oz) of them with milk, sugar substitute, almonds and fruit as desired.

Helpful Hint: If there are any leftovers, be sure to refrigerate them.

SMOKY BLACK BEAN SOUP (4 servings)
The wonderful flavour of smoked turkey permeates it. Look for smoked turkey legs in delicatessens.

1 tbsp rapeseed oil
1 onion, diced
2 cloves garlic, crushed
1 jalapeno pepper, seeded and minced
2 cans (2 x 410g/14oz) black beans, drained and rinsed
1.5 litres (3½ pints) chicken stock (low-fat, low-sodium)
1 smoked turkey leg (about 575g/1¼lb)
80g (2¾oz) tomato paste
2 green peppers, diced
1 tomato, seeded and diced
10g (½oz) chopped fresh coriander
60ml (2fl oz) light soured cream

1. In a large stockpot, heat the oil over a medium heat. Cook the onion, garlic and jalapeno pepper for about 3 minutes or until softened. Add the beans, stock, turkey leg and tomato paste. Bring to the boil; reduce the heat and simmer for about 1 hour or until the turkey begins to break apart.

2. Remove the turkey leg and set aside. Pour the soup into a blender in batches and purée it until smooth. Return it to the pot over a medium heat. Add the peppers and tomato and heat until steaming.

3. Meanwhile, remove the meat from the turkey leg and chop; add to the soup. Serve sprinkled with coriander and a dollop of soured cream.

VARIATIONS:
Ham option: You can substitute smoked ham or ham hock for the turkey leg.

OPEN-FACED CHICKEN REUBEN SANDWICH (4 servings)

This hefty sandwich used to be a big favourite when I worked in restaurants for the lunch crowd. It is also great for dinner served up with a hearty salad and fruit for dessert. Lightened up and packed with fibre and spiked with a tangy spread, this will keep you going for the rest of the evening.

Sandwich Spread:
110g (4oz) plain yoghurt
2 tsp balsamic vinegar
1 hard-boiled egg, finely chopped
2 tsp green olives, finely chopped
2 tsp red pepper, finely chopped
½ tsp Worcestershire sauce

4 slices stone-ground wholemeal high-fibre bread
375g (13oz) cooked chicken, chopped
200g (7oz) cabbage, shredded
1 tomato, sliced
4 slices light-style Swiss cheese
2 tsp non-hydrogenated spread or rapeseed oil

1. Sandwich Spread: In a small bowl, whisk together the yoghurt, balsamic vinegar, egg, olives, red pepper and Worcestershire sauce. Divide evenly among bread and spread. Top with chicken, cabbage and tomato. Lay one slice of cheese on each sandwich.

2. In a large ovenproof non-stick frying pan, melt the spread over a medium-high heat, or use rapeseed oil instead. Place the sandwiches in the frying

pan, in batches if necessary, and cook for about 5 minutes or until the bread is toasted. Place the frying pan in a 200°C, Gas 6, oven for about 5 minutes or until the cheese melts.

Helpful hint: You can pick up 2 cooked chicken legs at the supermarket and, once they are de-boned and the skin has been removed, you should have about 375g (13oz); or you could also use leftover roasted or grilled chicken or turkey.

CHILLED SPINACH AND WATERCRESS SOUP (4–6 servings)
This creamy soup makes a nice starter for a summer meal.

750 ml 1 ⅓ pts vegetable stock
1 x 200g baby leaf spinach, chopped
1 x 100g bag watercress, chopped
1 x 287ml carton buttermilk or 250ml (9fl oz) low-fat natural yoghurt
1 x 200g can water chestnuts, drained and chopped
4 tbsp half-fat crème fraiche or 0%-fat fromage frais
1 clove garlic, crushed
2 tbsp chopped fresh mint
½ tsp each sea salt and pepper

1. Bring the stock to a simmer in a large saucepan. Add the spinach and watercress and cook for 3 minutes or just until wilted. Remove from heat and cool slightly.

2. Stir in the buttermilk, water chestnuts, crème fraiche, garlic, mint and seasoning.

3. In blender or food processor, purée a quarter of the soup until smooth then stir back into the remaining soup. Chill for at least 2 hours before serving.

Storage: Keeps for up to 1 day in the fridge.

QUICK FISH STEAKS WITH TOMATO-CHICKPEA RELISH

(4 servings)

This recipe is so versatile, you can use fish, chicken, turkey or, my favourite, lamb chops! The slight sweetness of the relish complements the peppery bite of the fish. It's perfect served with basmati rice and green beans.

60ml (2fl oz) red-wine vinegar
2 tbsp chopped fresh thyme or 1 tsp dried
2 cloves garlic, crushed
2 tsp Dijon mustard
½ tsp pepper
4 tuna steaks

Tomato Chickpea Relish:
2 large tomatoes, deseeded and finely chopped
175g (6oz) chopped cooked chickpeas
40g (1½oz) finely chopped red pepper
40g (1½oz) finely chopped onion
5g (¼oz) chopped flat-leaf parsley
60ml (2fl oz) apple cider vinegar
1 tbsp sugar substitute
2 tsp pickling spice
1 pinch each salt and pepper

1. Tomato Relish: In a large bowl, stir together the tomatoes, chickpeas, red pepper, onion, parsley, vinegar, sugar substitute, pickling spice, salt and pepper. Let stand for 10 minutes.

2. In a large shallow dish, stir together the red-wine vinegar, thyme, garlic, mustard and pepper. Add the fish steaks and turn to coat. Let stand for 5 minutes.

3. Place the steaks on a greased grill over a medium-high heat and grill for about 8 minutes, turning once or until medium-rare or desired doneness. Serve with the relish.

VARIATIONS:
Yellow-light option: You can use 8 lean lamb chops in place of the fish fillets. Increase cooking time to 10 minutes for medium-rare.

Chicken option: You can use 4 chicken breasts, skinned, instead of the fish. Increase cooking time to about 25 minutes.

GRILLED FRUIT KEBABS WITH A LEMON-YOGHURT SAUCE

Here's a simple way to turn plain fruit into something special. You can add in a small amount of yellow-light pineapple.

Choose about 750g (1lb 10oz) total prepared weight from a mixture of green-light fruits:
Cubed pitted peaches, nectarines or plums
Seedless orange segments
Seedless grapes
Pitted sweet cherries

Yoghurt Sauce:
250g (9oz) low-fat natural yoghurt
4 tbsp sugar substitute
2 tbsp fresh lemon juice
2 tsp chopped fresh lemon balm or mint
2 tsp grated lemon zest
Lemon balm sprigs or mint sprigs

1. Thread the prepared fruits alternately on to 8 metal or soaked wooden skewers.

2. Make the yoghurt sauce – mix together the yoghurt, sugar substitute, lemon juice, chopped lemon balm or mint and lemon zest in a bowl.

3. Place the skewers on a greased grill pan over a medium-high heat. Grill 4 minutes per side or until fruit is warm and lightly browned.

4. Drizzle some of the sauce over the kebabs and serve the plates garnished with lemon balm sprigs or mint sprigs. Serve the rest of the sauce in a bowl for dipping.

DAY 7

HOMEY OATMEAL (4 servings)

*This hot breakfast is guaranteed to keep you feeling satisfied all morning.
You can vary the flavour by topping it with fresh fruit such as berries or
chopped apple.*

450ml (15fl oz) skimmed milk
325ml (11fl oz) water
1 tsp cinnamon
¼ tsp salt
150g (5oz) large-flake oats
25g (1oz) wheat germ
25g (1oz) chopped almonds
3 tbsp sugar substitute

In a large saucepan, bring the milk, water, cinnamon and salt to the boil.
Stir in the oats and wheat germ and return to the boil. Reduce the heat to
low and cook, stirring, for about 8 minutes or until the mixture has thickened. Stir in the almonds and sugar substitute.

TUSCAN WHITE-BEAN SOUP (4 servings)

*I first tried this country-style soup in Tuscany and immediately fell in love
with it. I serve this soup in deep Italian ceramic soup bowls and dream I'm
back in Tuscany.*

1 tbsp extra-virgin olive oil
1 onion, chopped
4 cloves garlic, crushed
1 carrot, chopped
1 celery stalk, chopped
4 fresh sage leaves or ½ tsp dried
1.5 litres (2½ pints) vegetable or chicken stock (low-fat, low-sodium)
2 cans (2 x 410g/14oz) cannellini or white kidney beans, drained and rinsed
320g (11oz) shredded kale
1 pinch each salt and pepper

1. In a large stockpot, heat the oil over a medium heat. Add the onion, garlic,
carrot, celery and sage and cook for 5 minutes or until softened.

2. Add the stock, beans, kale, salt and pepper, and cook, stirring occasionally,
for about 20 minutes or until the kale is tender.

ROASTED RED-PEPPER HUMMUS (about 700g /1½lb)

Serve this as a dip with raw veggies or as a spread for sandwiches or hamburgers. You could also enjoy it on its own in half a whole-wheat pitta with tomatoes and cucumber slices.

1 can (410g/14oz) chickpeas, drained and rinsed
50g (2oz) chopped roasted red peppers
25g (1oz) tahini
½ tsp ground cumin
½ tsp salt
2 tbsp extra-virgin olive oil
2 tbsp water
1 tbsp lemon juice
1 small clove garlic, crushed

In a food processor, pulse together the chickpeas, peppers, tahini, cumin and salt. With the food processor running, add the oil and water until it is very smooth. Pulse in the lemon juice and garlic.

VARIATIONS:
Sundried-tomato version: Omit the roasted red peppers. Use 10g (½oz) chopped sundried tomatoes that have been rehydrated in hot water and drained.

Roasted-vegetable hummus: Omit the roasted red peppers. Use 110g (4oz) chopped roasted vegetables.

Storage: Keep in an airtight container, refrigerated, for up to 2 weeks.

Helpful hint: Tahini is a sesame-seed paste that you can find in health-food shops and most supermarkets. It adds a great nutty flavour to the hummus.

CHICKEN TAGINE (4 servings)

The flavour of this Moroccan-inspired stew develops with time. So, make it a day ahead and reheat it for a satisfying mid-week meal served on a bed of basmati rice. Don't be frightened by the long list of ingredients. The first nine make up a spice rub.

3 cloves garlic, crushed
2 tsp grated fresh root ginger
1 tsp ground paprika
1 tsp ground cumin
½ tsp ground cinnamon
½ tsp turmeric
½ tsp ground black pepper
¼ tsp saffron strands, crushed finely
¼ tsp sea salt
4 skinless, boneless chicken breasts, about 125g (4½oz) each, cut in half lengthways
2 tsp olive oil
1 large onion, thinly sliced
1 x 410g can chickpeas, drained and rinsed
75g (3oz) dried apricots, sliced
25g (1oz) raisins
4 tbsp chopped fresh coriander
4 tbsp chopped fresh parsley
2 tbsp lemon juice
½ lemon, thinly sliced
4 tbsp chopped fresh mint

1. In a large bowl, mix together the garlic, ginger, paprika, cumin, cinnamon, turmeric, pepper, saffron and salt. Mix in the chicken rubbing the spice mixture well into the meat. Set aside for a few minutes.

2. In a large deep non-stick frying pan, heat the oil over a medium-high heat. Add the onion and cook until softened, about 5 minutes. Then add the chicken and brown on all sides, about 5 minutes.

3. Add about 500ml (18fl oz) water, the chickpeas, apricots, raisins, coriander, parsley, lemon juice and lemon slices. Bring to the boil then reduce the heat to a simmer, cover and cook for about 15–20 minutes or until chicken is firm and no longer pink inside. Garnish with chopped mint.

PECAN BROWNIES (16 brownies)

Brownies, you ask? That's right. These are packed with fibre and are absolutely scrumptious, so get baking!

1 can (410g/14oz) white or red kidney or black beans, drained and rinsed
120ml (4fl oz) skimmed milk
2 omega-3 eggs
50g (2oz) non-hydrogenated spread, melted
1 tbsp vanilla essence
12 tbsp sugar substitute
50g (2oz) wholemeal flour
50g (2oz) unsweetened cocoa powder
1 tsp baking powder
1 pinch salt
75g (3oz) chopped toasted pecan nuts

1. In a food processor, purée the beans until coarse. Add in the milk, eggs, spread and vanilla essence and purée until smooth, scraping down the sides a few times. Set it aside.

2. In a large bowl, combine the sugar substitute, flour, cocoa, baking powder and salt. Pour the bean mixture over the flour mixture. Stir to combine. Scrape the mixture into a greaseproof-paper-lined 20cm (8in) square baking pan, smoothing the top. Sprinkle it with pecans.

3. Bake in a 180°C, Gas 4, oven for about 18 minutes or until a skewer inserted into the centre comes out clean. Allow to cool on a rack.

Storage: Cover these brownies with cling film or store them in an airtight container for up to 4 days. They can also be frozen for up to 2 weeks.

8 The Green-Light Glossary

It's helpful to know a little about the most popular green-light foods, so here's a handy alphabetical summary. For a full green-light list, see Appendix I.

Apples
These are a real staple, and make a great snack or dessert. Unsweetened apple purée is ideal with cereals, or with cottage cheese as a snack.

Beans (legumes)
You can never get enough beans. These perfect green-light foods are high in protein and fibre and can supplement nearly every meal. Make bean salads or just add beans to any existing salad recipe to boost their protein and fibre. Add to soups, replace some of the meat in casseroles or add to meat-loaf recipes. Use as a side vegetable or as an alternative to potatoes, rice or pasta.

Check out the wide range of canned and frozen beans, but be careful with baked beans, however, as the sauce can be high-sugar and high-calorie. Check the label for reduced-sugar versions and watch the size of your serving.

Beans have a well-deserved reputation for creating 'firmness to the bite', so be patient until your body adapts – as it will – to your increased consumption.

Bread
Most breads are red-light except for coarse or stone-ground, 100% whole-wheat or wholemeal breads. Check labels carefully as the bread industry likes to confuse the unwary. The ideal wording is 'Stone-ground, 100% wholemeal'.

In order to qualify as green-light, breads must contain 2.5–3g of fibre per slice. Most bread is made from flour ground by steel rollers, which strip away the bran coating, leaving a very fine powder ideal for producing light, fluffy breads and pastries. Stone-ground flour, on the other hand, is coarser and retains more of its bran coating, so it is digested more slowly in your stomach.

Even with stone-ground, 100% wholemeal bread, watch your serving sizes, and use sparingly where you cannot avoid it, such as lunch in Phase I.

Cereals
You should only use large-flake or 'old-fashioned' porridge oats, oat bran or high-fibre cold cereals (10g fibre per serving or higher). Though these cereals might not seem that appealing in themselves, you can liven them up with fruit or fat-free yoghurt with sweetener. This way, you can change the menu daily. And sprinkle sweetener on your cereal if you need to, not sugar.

Cottage cheese
Low-fat or fat-free cottage cheese is an excellent low-fat, high-protein food. Add fruit to make a snack or add it to salads.

Eggs
Whole eggs are yellow-light – stick to egg whites in Phase I. When you move on to Phase II, the best option is omega-3-enriched eggs as omega-3 essential fatty acids are good for heart health.

Food bars
Most food or nutrition bars are a dietary disaster, high in carbohydrates and calories but low in protein. These bars are quick sugar fixes on the run. There are a few, such as Myoplex/Slim-Fast bars, that have a more equitable distribution of carbohydrates, proteins and fats. Look for 20–30g carbohydrates, 12–15g protein and 4–6g fat. This equals about 220 calories per 50g bar.

The serving size for a snack is one-half of a bar. Keep one in your office desk or your handbag for a convenient on-the-run snack.

In an emergency, I have been known to have one bar plus an apple and a glass of skimmed milk for lunch when a proper lunch break was impossible. This is OK in emergencies, but don't make a habit of it.

Grapefruit
One of the top-rated green-light foods. Eat as often as you like.

Hamburgers
These are acceptable but only with extra-lean minced beef that has 10% or less fat. If you're making your own (which is best), mix in some oat bran to reduce the meat content but keep the bulk. A better option would be to replace the beef with ground turkey or chicken breast, which is lower in fat. Keep the serving size at 110g (4oz). Use only half of a wholemeal bun and eat it open-faced.

Meat
The best green-light meats are skinless chicken and turkey breast, top/eye round beef, pork tenderloin, veal, deli cuts of lean ham and back bacon.

Milk
You should only use skimmed milk, to minimise your saturated (bad) fat intake. If you have trouble adjusting, then use semi-skimmed and slowly wean yourself off it. Milk is a terrific snack or meal supplement. I drink two glasses of skimmed milk a day, at breakfast and lunch. Low-fat plain (unsweetened) soya milk is an excellent alternative if you are lactose intolerant.

Nuts
A great source of 'good' fat, which is essential for your health. Add them to cereals, salads and desserts. Almonds are your best choice.

Oat bran
An excellent high-fibre additive to baking as a partial replacement for flour, or as a hot cereal, prepared like porridge.

Oranges
Whole or in segments, fresh oranges are excellent as snacks, on cereal and especially at breakfast. A glass of orange juice has $2\frac{1}{2}$ times as many calories as a whole orange, so avoid the juice and stick with the real thing.

Pasta
Though wholemeal and thicker pastas are best in Gi terms, most pastas are acceptable. There are two golden rules. First, do not overcook: it's important for the pasta to retain some 'firmness to the bite' (al dente, as the Italians say). Second, serving size: pasta is a side dish and should never occupy more than a quarter of your plate. It must not form the basis of the meal, as it most commonly does nowadays, with disastrous results for the waistline and hips.

Peaches/pears
These make terrific snacks, desserts or additions to breakfast cereal. Eat them fresh, or canned in juice or water (not syrup).

Porridge
If you haven't had porridge since you were a kid, now's the time to revisit it. Large-flake, or old-fashioned, porridge is the breakfast of choice, with the added heart benefit of lowering your cholesterol. I often have an oatmeal porridge snack with unsweetened apple purée and sweetener on the weekends.

Potatoes

The only form of potatoes that is acceptable, even on an occasional basis, when you're eating the Gi way, is boiled new potatoes. Limit quantity to two or three per serving.

New potatoes are low in starch, unlike larger, more mature potatoes that have been allowed to build up their starch levels. All other forms of potato – baked, mashed or fried – are strictly red-light.

Rice

The various types of rice have a wide range of Gi ratings, and most of them are red-light. The best rice is basmati or long grain, and brown is better than white. If rice is sticky, with the grains clumping together, don't use it. Similarly, don't overcook rice; the more it's cooked, the more glutinous and therefore unacceptable it becomes.

The rule, then, is to eat only slightly undercooked basmati rice (preferably brown), which is readily available at your supermarket.

Salads

You should include a side salad in your diet every day if possible. Salad provides both an important fibre and low-Gi nutritional boost to your meals. As acidic foods can reduce the Gi of your meals by slowing absorption, a vinaigrette dressing is an excellent complementary bonus to your meal.

Sweeteners

Despite an intensive misinformation campaign by the sugar lobby, sugar substitutes are completely safe and approved by all major government and health authorities worldwide. The sugar industry rightly saw these new products as a threat and has done its best to bad-mouth them. Silver Spoon, Hermesetas and Splenda® (or their generic counterparts) can all be substituted for sugar. These sweeteners are available in several forms – individual packets, granules, liquid and tablets. My preference is for sweeteners such as Splenda® that measure exactly the same as sugar by volume, i.e. 1 tbsp sugar equals 1 tbsp sweetener. Remember, it's measuring the equivalent of sugar by volume and not by weight.

If you are allergic to sweeteners, then fructose (fruit sugar, available from health-food stores and some supermarkets) is a better alternative than sugar. A herbal alternative called 'stevia' is acceptable if used in moderation, as no long-term studies on its usage are available.

If you are sweetening a beverage or ready-to-eat meal, simply use your own taste as a guide. If you are substituting for sugar in baking, follow the instructions on the box or check the manufacturer's website.

Yoghurt

'Diet' fruit-flavoured yoghurt with sweetener is a near-perfect green-light product. It's an ideal snack food on its own, or a flavourful addition to breakfast cereal – especially porridge oats – and to fruit for dessert. My fridge is always full of it, in half-a-dozen delicious flavours.

Note: All dairy products contain lactose, a natural sugar found in milk. That is why there are no completely sugar-free dairy products.

Yoghurt cheese

A wonderful substitute for cream in desserts or to finish off main dishes like chilli (see recipe on page 86).

9 Staying Power – Keeping Yourself Motivated

Food cravings, holidays and celebrations, vacations and flagging enthusiasm are all challenges to our commitment to healthy eating. But don't worry if, from time to time, you 'fall off the wagon', eating or drinking with friends and going outside the Gi programme. That's the real world and it's more important that you don't feel as though you're living in a straitjacket. I probably live about 90% within the programme and 10% outside – by choice.

These tips will help to keep you motivated, especially when your resolve starts flagging – as it inevitably will from time to time:

• Maintain a weekly progress log (see page 156). Nothing is more motivating than success.
• Set up a reward system. If you are trying to lose weight, buy yourself a small gift when you achieve a predetermined weight goal.
• Find a friend who will join the plan for mutual support.
• Avoid acquaintances and haunts that may encourage your old behaviours and eating habits. We all have them!
• Try adding what my wife calls a special 'spa' day to your week – a day when you are especially good with your programme. (This also gives you some extra credit in your weight-loss account to draw on when the inevitable relapse occurs.)
• Sign up for the free Gi Diet e-mail newsletter to learn from readers' experiences and keep up to date on the latest developments in diet and health (details on www.gidiet.co.uk).

FOOD CRAVINGS

What makes losing weight, or even just sticking to a healthy eating plan, particularly challenging is that we tend to enjoy and desire fattening and unhealthy foods such as chocolate, cakes, biscuits, ice cream, peanut butter, chips and so on. The most important thing to remember about cravings is that we're only human and it's natural to succumb to temptation every now and then. Don't feel guilty about it. If you 'cheat', you aren't totally blowing your healthy-eating plan. You're simply experiencing a temporary blip in your good eating habits. If you have a small piece of chocolate cake after dinner, or perhaps a beer with the guys while watching the game, make sure you savour the extravagance by eating or drinking slowly. Really enjoy it. Then get back on track in the morning with a green-light breakfast and stick to the straight and narrow for the next couple of weeks.

A friend of mine, who is a cardiologist, allows himself a few 'red days' a month. These are days when he knows he has strayed from the guidelines of the Gi Diet. To prevent red days from becoming a habit, he monitors them by marking them on his calendar. The Gi Diet itself will help prevent lapses in two key ways:

You will find that after you've been on the programme for a few weeks, you will have developed a built-in warning system: you won't feel good physically when you eat a red-light food because your blood sugar will spike and crash. You'll feel bloated, uncomfortable and lethargic, and you may even get a headache – a strong deterrent against straying into red-light territory.

Because you are eating three meals and three snacks daily, you won't feel hungry between meals. If you skip any, you will probably start longing for forbidden foods – so make sure you eat all the recommended meals and snacks every day.

So what should you do if a craving looks like getting the better of you, despite the diet's built-in security system? Well, you could try substituting a green-light food for the red-light food you're thinking about. If you want something sweet, try having fruit, 'diet' yoghurt, low-fat ice cream with no added sugar, one of the delicious low-Gi snacks in this book, one of my recommended food bars or a caffeine-free diet soft drink. If what you want is something salty and crunchy, try having a dill pickle or some dried chickpeas. Your craving for chocolate in Phase I may be alleviated with a chocolate-flavoured food bar, with a diet instant chocolate drink, a Chocolate Drop Cookie (see page 98) or Pecan Brownies (see page 107).

Sometimes, however, there isn't a likely substitute for the foods we miss. I have received many emails from readers who love peanut butter and say they cannot live without it. The thing to do here is to select the most nutritional product available – the natural kind that is made from peanuts only and has no additives such as sugar – and eat only a tablespoon of it once in a while. It's better to consume the good fats that are in peanuts than the red-light fillers that are found in other varieties of peanut butter. Don't be fooled into thinking the 'lite' versions are better for you – the amount of peanuts has been reduced and sugar and starch fillers have been added. And remember that the more red-light foods you consume, the more you will slow your progress in achieving your target BMI.

PARTIES AND CELEBRATIONS

We all know how much determination and gumption it takes to clear one's cupboards, go shopping and embark on an unfamiliar way of eating. That's why once we have managed to do all this, the last thing we want is for a holiday to come along and throw a wrench into our progress. Traditional festivals such as Christmas and Easter all have one thing in common: an abundance of food. Holidays are generally centred around traditional feasts and dishes. But even so, you don't have to throw the Gi guidelines out of the window. You can stay in the green and still have a fun and festive celebration.

If you host the event yourself, you will be able to decide what type of food is served. Think of what you would normally eat during the festivities and look for green-light alternatives. You can put on a completely green-light feast without your guests even realising. For example, if you usually have a roast turkey with bread-based stuffing for Christmas, have a roast turkey with wild or basmati rice stuffing instead. There is no shortage of green-light vegetables to serve as side dishes, and dessert can be elegant poached pears or a pavlova with berries.

If you celebrate the holiday at someone else's home, you will obviously have less control over the menu. Once seated at the table, survey the dishes and try to compose your plate as you would at home: vegetables on half the plate, rice or pasta on one quarter and a source of protein on the other.

Pass on the rolls and mashed potatoes – have extra vegetables instead. If you wish, you can allow yourself a concession by having a small serving of dessert. If you aren't particularly big on sweets, you might prefer to have a glass of wine instead. Try not to indulge in both.

Cocktail parties can also be fun, green-light occasions. Instead of alcohol, you can have a glass of mineral water with a twist of lemon or a diet caffeine-free soft drink. If you really would like an alcoholic beverage, have only one and try to choose the least red-light option. Red wine is your best bet, or a white-wine spritzer made half with wine and half with sparkling water. Be sure to consume any alcohol with food to slow down the rate at which you metabolise it. Beer has a very high-Gi rating, so that's a real concession. Have it if you really want it, but make sure it's only one. Other drinks are also high Gi and high calorie.

If you host the cocktail party yourself, you can make all the appetisers green-light. Have a cooked, sliced turkey as a centrepiece and offer lean sliced deli ham with a selection of mustards. Serve a variety of raw vegetables with a choice of low-fat dips and salsa. Hummus with wedges of whole-wheat pitta, smoked salmon or caviar on cucumber slices, crab salad and snow peas, chicken or beef skewers, meatballs made with extra-lean minced beef, and sashimi with soy sauce all make wonderful appetisers that everyone will enjoy. You can also provide bowls of nuts and olives, but remember to have only a few of each and don't linger nearby – it's too tempting to keep munching as you chat with your guests. Be sure to also serve a platter piled decoratively with a wide variety of green-light fruits.

If you are attending someone else's cocktail party, have a green-light meal before you go so you won't be tempted to eat too much. Then choose the low-Gi appetisers and enjoy your time with friends and family.

HOLIDAYS

Unless you are spending your holiday in a self-catering cottage or apartment, going away on holiday usually means having to eat all your meals at restaurants. But it's not terribly difficult to put the Gi guidelines into practice when dining out, as you've seen in Chapter 5.

And remember to avoid the Continental breakfasts offered in some hotels. They are generally made up of red-light foods and offer little in the way of nutrition. One option for breakfast is to buy your own fruit, green-light cereals and milk at a supermarket and have breakfast in your hotel room.

Just because you are on holiday doesn't mean you shouldn't continue to eat three meals and three snacks daily. Pack some green-light snacks to take with you, such as food bars, nuts and any other non-perishables. Once there, you can buy 'diet' yoghurts, fruit and low-fat cottage cheese to snack on.

If you are driving to your destination, your only option along the way may be fast food. If you can, pack some green-light meals and snacks to take with you, so you won't have to stop to eat.

10 Exercise

EXERCISE VERSUS DIET

Although exercise is very important, you need to remember that diet has far more impact on weight loss than exercise does. You can spend an hour on the treadmill and expend only 250 calories, which you can put right back on again if you eat half a large muffin on the way home. To give you some idea of how much exercise is required to lose just 1lb of weight, look at the following table:

EFFORT REQUIRED TO LOSE 1LB OF FAT		
	9-stone person	11-stone person
Walking (4mph, briskly)	53 miles/85km	42 miles/67km
Running (8min/mile)	36 miles/58km	29 miles/46km
Cycling (12–14mph)	96 miles/154km	79 miles/127km
Sex (moderate effort)	79 times	64 times

This is clearly unrealistic for most people. So during Phase I, the weight loss phase, diet will probably account for 90 per cent of your weight loss. Any exercise will help, but diet should be your principal focus.

However, exercise is an important contributor to maintaining your desired weight. For example, if you were to walk briskly for half an hour a day, seven days per week, you would burn up calories equalling twenty pounds of fat per year.

For women past the menopause, weight-bearing exercise is one way to counteract osteoporosis and the risk of fractures. And for families, exercising together – biking, skiing, whatever you enjoy – not only helps control weight but is also a way to enjoy each other's company.

And if that's not reason enough to get moving, exercise is fantastic for all-round health.

WHY EXERCISE?

Regular exercise will:
• Help you to lose weight and maintain a healthy weight;
• Dramatically reduce your risk of heart disease, stroke, diabetes and osteoporosis;
• Improve your mental well-being and boost your self-esteem;
• Help you to sleep better.

Exercise works in exactly the same way as diet to reduce or control weight. The more energy (calories) you expend than you take in, the more your body will use up your energy reserve (fat) to make up the shortfall. Exercise burns calories. In fact, every action you perform uses calories. So, climbing the stairs instead of taking the lift to your office, getting off the bus a stop or two early, or parking as far away as possible from the shopping centre or supermarket entrance will require extra activity over your normal routine and thereby consume extra calories.

As we noted earlier, if you were to walk briskly for half an hour a day, you would lose 20lbs a year automatically. How come? Well, a brisk half-hour walk consumes approximately 200 extra calories. Multiply that by 365 days and you get 73,000 calories, or 20lbs/1 ½ stone (1 pound = 3,600 calories).

Note: the 30-minute (2.5km) walk that burns 200 calories is based on a 10st 10lbs (68kg) person. Heavier people will burn more calories in thirty minutes, and lighter people will burn fewer. A 14st 4lbs (90kg) person will burn 220 calories, a 9st 9lbs (60kg) person 175 calories. And the more briskly you walk, the more calories you will consume.

Exercise has two further benefits on weight loss and control.

Exercise increases your metabolism – the rate at which you burn up calories – even after you've finished exercising. In other words, the benefits stay with you all day. Exercise in the morning is particularly beneficial as it sets the pace for your metabolism for the day.

Exercise builds muscle mass. Though regular exercise will help minimise muscle loss, it is resistance exercises that actually build muscle mass. Resistance exercises are those where weights, elastic bands or hydraulics are used for muscles to pull or push against. Most of you are probably cringing at the thought of sweating body builders doing endless painful workouts with massive barbells and other daunting equipment. It does not have to be like that. A few simple exercises will do wonders to tone and restore those flabby muscles.

GETTING MOVING

Getting started is one of the hardest challenges. Many of us are put off from taking the first steps by believing exercise is painful, time consuming, or just plain boring.

So let's look at the three excuses head on. First, there's the pain or discomfort excuse. This probably comes from an experience where you've tried to do too much too soon. The world's lofts are full of exercise equipment purchased in a moment of excessive enthusiasm. A few weeks later, aching muscles, a sore bottom and burning lungs have relegated that exercise bike or other exotic machine to the deep, dark storeroom where we put things that 'may be useful later'.

Does that sound familiar?

To avoid pain, you must start small and work yourself up. Start with walking and if you start gently and increase gradually, it is pain-free.

The second objection is lack of time. There are 336 thirty-minute blocks of time each week. Take 2%, or seven, of these blocks and use one each day. This can hardly be an unreasonable allocation of your time, especially when you consider the benefits: a slimmer, fitter, healthier you! Thirty minutes a day should be your target, though I know that many of you will want to increase this allocation once you feel the remarkable improvements that such a modest time commitment can bring.

As far as what time of day you should exercise is concerned, there are two clear camps: those who are at their best first thing in the morning and those who warm up during the day to hit their peak in the evening. So choose your best time – either bounding out of bed to greet the dawn or exercising away accumulated tensions at the end of the day.

Many people find that as their level of fitness increases, they sleep better and wake up feeling more refreshed, taking less time to drag themselves from bed. This in itself frees up more time for exercise, resulting in even less of a draw upon your day. Once you lose a bit of weight, being active will be something you crave and delight in. So stick with it – the fun will kick in eventually.

The third objection to exercise is boredom. I am very sympathetic to this one. While some exercises like jogging, walking and bicycling are, by their outdoor nature, rarely boring – unless people, and what they do and where they live, are of no interest to you – cold, damp winters can be a disincentive.

There is no doubt that working alone is more of a challenge. Many people use fitness clubs for both the motivation ('I've paid my fee, so I'd better use it') as well as the social interaction and mutual encouragement.

I chose the spare bedroom, as there was no gym nearby. My solution to the inherent boredom came via an ancient TV abandoned by the children as they left the nest, and an early 'replay only' video. I recorded those shows and films that ran between midnight and 6 a.m. on the family video, and they provided my entertainment. I pedalled and skied my way through James Bond movies, build-your-own-cottage shows and Jacques Cousteau under-sea documentaries. There was never a boring moment. In fact, I sometimes became so engrossed in the shows that I exercised far beyond my scheduled time allocation. A little ingenuity (which could be as simple as loading your favourite tunes on your iPod) can certainly help make workouts more interesting.

TYPES OF EXERCISE

Before we go any further, we should define exactly what we mean by exercise. There are three basic types of exercise, each working in a synergistic relationship with the others.

Aerobic
The objective of aerobic exercise is to get your heart and lungs working harder. Aerobic exercise (walking, jogging, biking, swimming, hiking and so on) will have the most impact on your overall weight and health.

Strength training
As we move into middle age and beyond, strength exercise is particularly important because of the steady reduction in muscle mass that accompanies ageing. Starting at the age of 25, the body loses 2% of its muscle mass each decade, a process that accelerates to 6–8% as we move into our senior years.

By exercising muscles on a regular basis, the loss can be minimised or reversed. This is because the larger your muscles, the more energy (calories) they use. So whether at work or at rest, increased muscle mass helps you lose or maintain your weight.

Try a few strength exercises, concentrating on the larger muscle groups – your legs, arms and upper chest. These are the muscles that will give you the biggest bang by burning up the most calories. The resistance exercises should complement your other regular exercise regimen, not replace it. Committing to both types of exercise will produce far better results than either one alone. Resistance exercises are best done every other day, leaving time for your muscles to recuperate.

Resistance-training equipment can range from the complex and expensive to a £5 rubber resistance band. Home gyms, with prices that begin at a couple of hundred pounds, are a popular option. For most people, however, there are cheaper, simpler methods, such as a set of free weights or (my own preference) rubber resistance bands such as Dyna-Band. These resistance bands and weights are available at many fitness-exercise-equipment retailers.

Flexibility

This is a significant issue as we age and lose flexibility in our joints, tendons and ligaments. Loss of flexibility reduces our ability to do either aerobic or strength training, both of which depend on healthy joints and tissues. In older people, this loss of flexibility can lead to falls and hip fractures. So although stretching may seem like a 'frill', it is central to the whole fitness picture.

Stretching exercises can give you noticeable results very quickly. Within just a week, you can increase your flexibility by over 100%. Both aerobic and strength training can actually make you less flexible if you don't stretch those muscle ligaments and tendons. That's why you always see athletes warming up and down with stretching exercises. So always include stretching, whether a simple set of muscle stretches or a yoga or T'ai Chi session, in your exercise programme.

Now let's look at your exercise options.

OUTDOOR ACTIVITIES

Walking

This is by far the simplest and, for most people, the easiest exercise programme to start and maintain. You don't need any special clothing or equipment, except a pair of comfortable cushioned shoes or trainers. Walking is rarely boring since you can keep changing routes and watch the world go by. Walk with an older son or daughter for company and mutual support, or go solo and commune with nature and your own thoughts. If you have a child in a pushchair, you can set a brisk pace that way. A great idea is to incorporate your walking into your daily commute to work. I get off the bus three stops early on my way to and from work. Those three stops are equal to about 2.5 kilometres (1½ miles), so I'm walking about 5 kilometres (3 miles) per day! If you drive to work, try parking your car about 2.5 kilometres (1½ miles) away and walk to your job. You may even find cheaper parking further out. However, start with just one stop early (or the equivalent) and work up. Who knows – distance permitting, you may eventually be able to walk to work. Think of the savings in petrol and parking fees!

For adults, 30 minutes a day 7 days a week should be your target. If you add 1 hour-long walk on the weekend, you can take a day off during the week. Remember we're talking about brisk walking, not speed walking nor ambling along. The pace should increase your heart and breathing rates, but never to the point where you lack the breath to carry on a conversation.

Hiking

Another variation on walking is cross-country hiking. Because this usually involves different kinds of terrain, especially hills and valleys, you use up more calories, about 50% more than for brisk walking. The reason for this is that you expend considerably more energy going uphill.

Hiking is fun, too, and is an especially good motivator for the whole family. It's an excuse for a special excursion out of town and for some adventure that can include every age, even a baby in a backpack. The only caveat is to choose a route that offers a variety of loops, from short to long. If your younger children flag, you can make your hikes suitable to the limits of the smallest. One way to satisfy everyone's level of fitness is to take turns: while you are with 'slow pack' – one parent plus the kids – your partner jogs or walks ahead, then loops back to join you and change over. This gives everyone a satisfying outing.

Jogging

This exercise is similar to walking, but more care is needed with footwear to protect joints from damage. The advantage of jogging over walking is that it approximately doubles the number of calories burned in the same period of time – 400 calories for jogging versus 200 for brisk walking over a thirty-minute period. While walking, try jogging for a few yards and see if this is for you. It will get your heart rate up, which is great for heart health. The heart is basically a muscle, and like all muscles it thrives on being exercised – in general, the more the better. If jogging is for you, then this could arguably be the simplest and most effective method of exercise, as it uses personal time efficiently, can be done any time, anywhere, and is inexpensive.

Cycling

Like walking, jogging and hiking, cycling is a fun way to burn up those calories, and it is almost as effective as jogging . And for people with low-back or knee problems, it can be preferable. Other than the cost of the bike, it's inexpensive and can be done almost anywhere and any time. It can also be done indoors during winter months with a stationary bike. Cycling offers another good change of pace from your regular routine. I find it gives me a chance to visit all sorts of communities outside my normal walking range.

Sports

Although most sports are terrific calorie burners, they usually cannot be part of a regular routine and are no substitute for a 5–7-day-a-week regular schedule. But they can provide a boost to your regular fitness-and-exercise programme.

Most sports require other people, equipment and facilities. Such popular sports as tennis, basketball, soccer, softball and golf (no golf buggy, please) are excellent additions to a basic exercise programme.

Other outdoor activities

Rollerblading, ice skating, skiing (especially cross-country), and swimming are good alternatives to, or changes of pace from, any of the above activities. They are similar to cycling in terms of energy consumption.

INDOOR ACTIVITIES

If you want to exercise indoors, the alternatives are either to organise a home gym or join a fitness club. The advantage of clubs is that they offer a wide range of sophisticated equipment, with instruction and advice from staff. Clubs are also social, and some people find they need group motivation to work out with enthusiasm. Many local authorities also offer special programmes including some for the elderly, new mothers and those with special needs, and may provide subsidies for people who can't afford the fees. Many community centres offer free fitness classes, too.

If a fitness club isn't convenient or those Lycra-clad young things make you feel intimidated, you can always set up your exercise area at home. The best and least expensive piece of equipment is a stationary bike. The latest models work on magnetic resistance rather than the old friction strap around the flywheel. This gives a smoother action, with better tension adjustment. Most important, they are quiet, which is crucial if you want to be able to listen to music or watch TV. You can easily pay thousands for a bike with all the fancy trimmings, but the £125–£150 machines will work fine. Just be sure you choose one that has smooth, adjustable tension, then pop in that late-night movie or your favourite soap and get pedalling. You'll be amazed how quickly the minutes fly by: 20 minutes on the bike consumes the same number of calories as 30 minutes of brisk walking.

If biking is not for you, try a treadmill. These can be expensive, and beware of the lower-end models that cannot take the pounding. Expect to pay about £500 and upwards. Make sure the incline of the track can be raised and lowered for a better workout.

Both treadmills and bikes can simulate outdoor walking, jogging, hiking or biking in the comfort of your own home. I use both of these machines but have added a cross-country ski machine, which has the advantage of working the upper body as well. Ski machines are generally less expensive than treadmills, but they cost more than stationary bikes. They also burn a higher number of calories (similar to jogging) because they use the arms and shoulders as well as the legs. It's almost the perfect all-body-workout machine.

There are several other specialised options, such as stair-climber machines, elliptical walkers and rowing machines, but they're not for everyone. They are also quite expensive, so make sure you try them out first at a fitness club or with a co-operative retailer before parting with your money.

Pilates

I've recently become a Pilates enthusiast. Originally, it was recommended by my physiotherapist to strengthen my back and prevent my disc problem from recurring. However, this very precise system of exercises does a lot more than just that. It's a series of floor exercises – no equipment needed – that both strengthen and stretch your muscles, especially the core muscles in your back and around your waist, which are essential for good posture. It's great for any level of fitness and at any age, and it is much less boring than step classes or other gym routines.

Yoga and T'ai Chi

Yoga comes in different styles now – Hatha, Kundalini, Kripalu, Ashtanga, Bikram and others. If you're new to yoga, the best choice is Hatha, which teaches you simple postures that will keep you supple, offer relaxation techniques and improve your breathing and circulation. Ashtanga is trendy nowadays, but it is more aerobic and demanding. Kundalini focuses on energising breathing techniques and meditation. But in any form, this ancient practice has much to offer, especially to anyone taking up exercise in middle age.

Another Eastern discipline, T'ai Chi is gentle and promotes flexibility, balance and energy. It features a series of flowing postures, done standing, that many people like to practise early in the morning, out of doors. It keeps the joints and tendons supple, and offers a peaceful, revitalising form of activity that can carry you into old age. With both T'ai Chi and yoga, there are a number of instructional DVDs or videos available for those who want to learn or practise at home.

As this is a book on nutrition, not exercise, I have not included any exercises for either stretching or strength training, particularly as there are a great number of excellent books on the subject. Check your local bookstore. Or you can consult the Web for free. For example, check out the BBC website (go to: www.bbc.co.uk/health/healthy-living/fitness).

Don't despair if you fall off the exercise – or diet – wagon now and then. The mistake most people make is that one wrong move makes them feel so bad that they give up. You don't have to be that hard on yourself. If you're living on the programme 90% of the time, you will still successfully lose weight, or not put it on if you are 'maintaining'.

Note: Most experts support the notion that any extra activity is better than none at all. I have no argument with that, but experience shows that if people start substituting washing the car or throwing the ball for the dog as alternatives to a regular brisk exercise programme, then the programme does not work. By all means garden, wash the windows or whatever else you like, but please do not fool yourself into thinking that this will have a significant impact on a weight-loss or maintenance programme.

The next step:

• Select an exercise that suits you. The fastest way to abandon an exercise programme is to do something you don't enjoy. It is best to select an exercise that uses the largest muscle groups, that is, the legs, abdominals and lower back. These burn more calories because of their sheer size. Walking, jogging and biking are excellent choices.

• Set goals and keep a record. An exercise log (see Appendix VII) is included to help keep you on track. Put it on the fridge or in the bathroom.

• Get support from family and friends. If possible, find a like-minded exercise buddy so you have support.

• Check with your doctor to ensure that she/he supports your plan.

11 Phase II

Phase II of the Gi Diet is for people who are at their target weight. If you've done this by losing weight through sticking to the principles of Phase I, congratulations! You kept at it and now you're reaping the benefits in terms of looking and feeling great.

You can now ease up a bit on limiting portion and serving sizes and start adding some yellow-light foods to your diet.

Of course, Phase II is also the danger zone, the stage when most diets go off the rails. And, frankly, when I take a close look at what many of these diets expect you to live on, I can understand why people can't stick to them for long.

The truth is you can lose weight on virtually any diet. Yes, it may be bad for your health and you may be half-starving, but you will drop the pounds if you manage to stick to it. The problem is that many diets – unlike the Gi Diet – are completely unsustainable. And, as I explained in Chapter 3, research tells us that there are three fundamental reasons why: the diets are too complicated, leave people feeling hungry, feeling unwell because of dietary imbalances – or a combination of the three.

The reality is that, with some modifications, the Gi Diet is your diet for life. But this isn't a hardship, because the Gi Diet was designed to give you a huge range of healthy choices, so you won't feel hungry, bored or unsatis- fied. By now, you will know how to navigate your green-light way around the supermarket aisles, you will know how to decipher food labels, and the colour coding of foods will be second nature. But the strangest thing may be that you are not even tempted to revert to your old ways. If you should fall prey to a double cheeseburger, you will be dismayed at how heavy, sluggish and ungratified you feel afterwards. You will be too attached to your new lightness and levels of energy to abandon them.

It may be hard to believe, but when I reached my target weight after losing twenty-two pounds, I had to make a conscious effort to eat more in order to avoid losing more weight. In Phase II, you must eat more than you did during the weight-loss portion of the diet in order to maintain your new weight. Remember the equation: food energy (calories) eaten must equal energy expended (used) to keep weight stable.

But I do have a few words of caution. You will require considerably less calories than you did before you started the diet because your body has become accustomed to doing with fewer calories and has to a certain extent adapted. Also, your metabolism has become more efficient, and your body has learned to do more with fewer calories than in its old spendthrift days. For example, if you lost 10 per cent of your body weight, you now require 10 per cent fewer calories.

Keep these two developments in mind when you head into Phase II. Your eyes may indeed be bigger than your stomach.

Try serving yourself slightly larger portion sizes or adding foods from the yellow-light category to your meals. Continue to monitor your weight each week, and if you start to gain, cut down a bit on the yellow-light foods; if you continue to lose, eat a bit more; if your weight remains stable, you've reached that magic balance and this is how you will eat for the rest of your life. You'll know what your body needs and you won't have to weigh yourself so often. You'll experience none of those hypoglyacemic lows and will no longer crave junk food. And you'll be able to cheat once in a while without gaining any pounds. You will be in control of your weight.

So add a few more calories, but don't go berserk, and remember to make yellow-light foods the exception rather than the rule. This way, you will keep the balance between the calories you're consuming and the calories you're expending – and that is the secret to stable weight.

Here are some ideas for how you could alter the way you eat in Phase II:

Breakfast
• Increase cereal serving size, e.g. from 50–75g (2–3oz) porridge.
• Add one of the yellow-light fruits – a banana or apricots – to your cereal.
• Add a slice of 100% whole-grain toast and a pat of non-hydrogenated spread.
• Double up on the sliced almonds on cereals.
• Enjoy an extra slice of back bacon.
• Have a glass of juice now and then.
• And you can now go caffeinated in the coffee department, if you like. But try to keep it to one cup a day.

Lunch
I suggest you continue to eat lunch as you did in Phase I. This is the one meal that contained some compromises in the weight-loss portion of the programme since it is a meal that most of us buy each day.

Dinner
• Add another boiled new potato (from two or three to three or four).
• Increase the rice or pasta serving by up to 50 per cent.
• Have a 175g (6oz) steak instead of your regular 110g (4oz).
• Enjoy a lean cut of lamb or pork.
• Add a slice of high-fibre bread or crispbread.
• Try a cob of sweet corn with a dab of non-hydrogenated margarine.
• Eat a few more olives and nuts.
• Have a glass of red wine with dinner.

Snacks
• Have some light microwave popcorn (the maximum serving is 1/3 of a packet).
• Indulge in a square or two of bittersweet, high cocoa (70%) chocolate.
• Eat a banana.
• Enjoy a scoop of low-fat ice cream or frozen yoghurt.

Alcohol
The other good news in Phase II is that a daily glass of wine, preferably red and with dinner, is not only allowed, it's encouraged! Red wine is particularly rich in flavonoids, and when it is drunk in moderation, it has a demonstrable benefit in reducing the risk of heart attack and stroke.

This requires discipline, though. Just because one glass is beneficial, it doesn't mean that two or three is even better for you. Immoderate drinking undoes any health benefits, and alcohol is always calorific. One glass of wine (150ml/5floz maximum) provides the optimum benefit. Apart from red wine, keep your consumption of alcohol to a minimum.

What about beer? Well, unfortunately for all us beer aficionados, beer has an exceptionally high-Gi rating due to its malt content. Still, I do enjoy an occasional pint. Real discretion is required here. If you do drink alcohol, always have it with a meal. Food slows down the absorption of alcohol, thereby minimising its impact.

Chocolate
This rich, luscious treat is the first thing all you chocoholics will want to incorporate back into your diet. And you can. Some chocolate – the right sort of chocolate, in the right amounts – is acceptable. Most chocolate contains too much saturated fat and sugar, which keeps it deep in the red-light zone. You need to choose chocolate with a high-cocoa content (a minimum of 70 per cent), because it delivers more chocolate intensity per ounce, and have only a square or two every once in a while. A couple of squares, nibbled slowly or dissolved in the mouth, are all you'll need to enjoy the taste and get the fix you need.

12 The Gi Diet and Health

People are getting more and more clued up about the health problems associated with being overweight or obese, as well as the huge impact that the food you eat has on your risk of illness, and your general well-being.

This is good – we have good reason to be concerned!

The fatter you are, the more likely you are to suffer a heart attack or stroke, to develop diabetes or to increase your risk for many cancers. And as we've clearly seen, your choice of foods and the quantity you consume will be the key determinant in how much you weigh.

Foods are fuel and a source of pleasure, too, but food can also have a biochemical effect on us that's as powerful as any drug. Everything we eat affects our health, well-being and emotional state, and this happens four or five times a day. Most of the time, we're looking for the pleasure angle rather than biochemistry. Imagine if we went to the medicine cabinet and chose our drugs the same way! The right foods can help you lose and maintain your weight, protect your health, extend your lifespan, give you more energy, and make you feel good and sleep better.

This is because food also affects health through the types of proteins, fats and carbohydrates we consume. The right choice can reduce your risk of heart disease, diabetes, prostate and colon cancers and Alzheimer's. Making the right choices is the principal theme of the Gi Diet. In this chapter, we will examine each of these major health issues and show you how to make the right choices to reduce your risk and improve your odds against these deadly diseases.

Eating the Gi way can reduce your risk of:

• Obesity (including central obesity – fat around your belly, the unhealthiest place to store it)
• Heart disease
• Stroke
• Diabetes
• Cancer
• Alzheimer's
• Arthritis

Obesity and central obesity

Being overweight is unhealthy, but even more important than the extra pounds you carry is where you carry them. It's much worse for your health to store fat around your middle – the so-called apple shape – than around your hips, thighs and bottom – the proverbial pear shape.

The beer belly

A beer belly, or 'apple shape', is not just an inert lump of fat. If you think that it just sits there, minding its own business and doing no harm, you'd be wrong. The most alarming medical news about fat, which runs contrary to conventional wisdom, is that it is not just a passive accumulator of energy stores and extra baggage. Rather, your fat is an active, living part of your body. In fact, this 'beer belly organ' behaves very much like any of our other body organs, such as the liver, heart or kidney, once it has formed sufficient mass.

But, unlike your other organs, this beer belly is actively undermining your body's health by pumping out a dangerous combination of free fatty acids and proteins. This causes out-of-control cell proliferation, which is directly associated with the growth of malignant cancerous tumours. In other words, fat seems to spur the growth of cancer, when those cells are present.

Body fat also creates inflammation, which is linked to atherosclerosis (clogged arteries), the principal cause of heart disease and stroke. And if that wasn't bad enough, body fat also increases insulin resistance, which can lead to type 2 diabetes.

In fact, these fat tissues have many characteristics of a huge tumour. The thought of that might help encourage many fence sitters to start doing something about that excess weight.

Heart disease and stroke

These are the two biggies. Heart disease and stroke account for about 40% of all deaths in England and Wales. Remarkably, this is evidence of progress. Twenty years ago, the figure was close to 50 per cent.

The good news is that advances in surgery, drug therapies and emergency services have saved many lives. The bad news is that twice as many deaths could have been averted if only we had reduced our weight, exercised regularly and quit smoking. Though the smoking rate for adults has dropped sharply (unfortunately, we cannot say the same for teens), we are eating more and exercising less, leading inevitably to a more obese and unhealthy population. It's been calculated that if we led even a moderate lifestyle, we could halve the carnage from these diseases.

Though heart disease, like most cancers, is primarily a disease of old age, nearly half of those who suffer heart attacks are under the age of sixty-five.

A familiar refrain that I have heard many times is, 'Why worry? If I have a heart attack, today's medicine will save me.' It might well save you from immediate death, but what most people do not realise is that the heart is permanently damaged after an attack. The heart cannot repair itself because its cells do not reproduce in the way that other organs do. (Ever wonder why you cannot get cancer of the heart? That's the reason.) After the damage sustained during a heart attack, the heart has to work harder to compensate – but it never can. It slowly degenerates under this stress, and patients finally 'drown' as blood circulation fails and the lungs fill with liquid. Congestive heart failure is a dreadful way to die, so make sure you do everything you can to avoid having a heart attack in the first place.

The simple fact is that many heart attacks could have been prevented by a healthy diet. Maintaining a sensible weight is crucial, too – the more over-weight you are, the more likely you are to suffer a heart attack or stroke.

I'm not going to dwell on the complexities of the science of nutrition and how it affects your heart and circulation; it's the outcome of this science that's important. However, a little science is helpful to understand the role and importance of both hypertension and cholesterol.

The two key factors linking heart disease and stroke to diet are hypertension (high blood pressure) and cholesterol.

Hypertension
Excess weight has a major bearing on blood pressure, which in turn can trigger life-threatening consequences. A Canadian study found that obese adults, aged eighteen to fifty-five, had a five- to thirteen-times greater risk of hypertension.

Why should we care? Hypertension is one of the harbingers of both heart attack and stroke. Think of the circulatory system as a huge system of stretchy tubes, containing fluid (blood) that is pumped around the body under pressure. With hypertension, there is too much stress on the arterial system, which causes it to age and deteriorate too rapidly. This eventually leads to arterial damage, blood clots and a heart attack or stroke.

In simple terms, a blockage in an artery to the heart triggers a heart at-tack (not enough blood and oxygen reach the heart), and a blockage in an artery going to or in the brain will cause a stroke (an area of the brain is starved of oxygen, and suffers damage or tissue death).

A recent study demonstrated that a lower-fat diet, coupled with a sizable increase in fruits and vegetables (eight to ten servings a day) lowered blood pressure. The moral: lose weight and eat more fruits and vegetables to help reduce your blood-pressure levels.

Cholesterol

Cholesterol has a bad reputation, but we need to understand its role more clearly. Cholesterol itself is essential to your body's metabolism, and we can't live without it, but high levels of cholesterol in the blood contribute to the plaque that builds up in your arteries, eventually causing blockage.

To make things more complicated, there are two forms of cholesterol: HDL (the good kind) and LDL (the bad). The idea is to boost HDL while suppressing LDL. (One way to remember the difference: HDL is 'Heart's Delight Level', and LDL is 'Leads to Death Level'.)

So we need to know what pushes the LDL levels up into the danger zone. The culprit? Saturated fat. The kind that turns solid at room temperature – cheese and butter are typical examples. This is also the fat that creates the 'marbling' effect in a tasty steak and makes bacon sizzle in the pan. Whole milk is high in saturated fat, and it's also hidden in crackers and pretzels.

Fortunately, not all fats are villains when it comes to our cholesterol levels. We have an ally in the form of the unsaturated fats. Not only do polyunsaturated and monounsaturated fats work to lower LDL levels, some of them actually boost HDL. So the no-fat diet is not a good idea. Instead, make sure that the right sort of fat is part of what you eat. (For the full picture on fats, see Chapter 1.)

In a nutshell:

Hypertension puts more stress on the arterial system, causing it to age and deteriorate more rapidly, contributing to arterial damage, blood clots, and heart attack or stroke.

High cholesterol is the key ingredient in the plaque that can build up in your arteries, eventually cutting off the supply of blood to your heart (causing heart attack) or your brain (leading to stroke).

The Gi Diet is the way to lower your blood pressure, control your cholesterol, and reduce your risk of cardiovascular disease.

Diabetes

Diabetes is the kissing cousin of heart disease in that more people die from heart complications arising from diabetes than from diabetes alone. In the UK 1.8 million people have the disease (more than 150 million world-wide) and these figures are increasing at an astonishing rate. It is predicted that, in the UK alone, another 1.2 million people will be diagnosed with diabetes over the next 5 years. The rates are skyrocketing – it's a real time-bomb situation.

The most common form of diabetes is called Type 2 diabetes. It used to be called Adult Onset diabetes as well, because it was rarely diagnosed in anyone below 40, but now so many younger people and children are developing diabetes that the name had to be changed.

The principal causes of the type 2 diabetes are obesity and lack of exercise, and the current epidemic is strongly correlated with the obesity trend. The fact that we are a culture in love with sugar contributes, too.

Now diabetics themselves are being advised that eating a low-Gi diet releases sugar more slowly into the bloodstream and helps stabilise blood-sugar levels, which, in turn, helps them control their diabetes. Eating the Gi way also helps them to lose weight, which also aids blood-sugar control.

Preventing diabetes, however, is far preferable to managing it. Since obesity and poor blood-sugar control are at the root of this condition, what more reason do you need to get right into your Gi Diet and exercise plan, and get those excess pounds off!

Diabetes and the obesity epidemic

The most dramatic illustration of this link I've seen is in Canada's Native population, where in some communities diabetes affects nearly half the adult population. Before the Europeans colonised North America, the Native peoples lived in a state of feast or famine. When there was an abundance of food, plant or animal, it was stored in the body as fat. In lean times, such as winter, the body depleted these fat supplies. As a result, their bodies developed a 'thrift gene'. Those who stored and utilised their food most effectively (i.e. they put on weight easily) were the survivors – a classic Darwinian exercise in survival of the fittest.

But when you took away the need to hunt or to harvest food and replaced it with a trip to the supermarket whenever food is required, the result was inevitable: a massive increase in obesity and, with it, diabetes.

Cancer

Every year, the evidence accumulates that your weight and your diet are critical risk factors for most forms of cancer. Being overweight has also been linked to cancer. Diets high in animal fats (saturated fats), such as the low-carb, high-protein regimes that have been popular recently, are also directly associated with increased vulnerability to breast, colon and prostate cancers. On the other hand, people who eat more fresh vegetables, fruits and whole grains seem to have a lower risk of developing these cancers. The American Institute for Cancer Research recommends that people eat a predominantly plant-based diet that includes a variety of vegetables, fruits and grains – the Gi Diet in a nutshell.

Breast and prostate cancer

Just as a low-saturated-fat diet can help protect women from developing breast cancer, a diet low in saturated fat has been shown to offer protection to men from prostate cancer, a disease which is even more pervasive among older men. Eating too much red meat puts men at higher risk of both prostate and colon cancer.

A diet low in animal fats and high in fresh fruits and vegetables – such as the Gi Diet – is a breast- and prostate-friendly diet.

Alzheimer's

Over the past few years, there has been a steady flow of research studies linking Alzheimer's and dementia with diet. A recent US study showed a 40% increase in Alzheimer's disease for those who ate a high-saturated-fat diet. In addition, anyone with a body mass index of 30 or higher is two-and-a-half times more likely to develop dementia. (Note: This study was based on data from more than 7,000 men. We don't know the implications for women.)

Alcohol, salt and refined carbohydrates were also associated with risk. On the upside, a diet rich in oily fish, such as salmon, sardines, mackerel and herring, can help prevent Alzheimer's. It seems that omega-3 oil and the vitamin E found in these fish are the helpful agents.

Many studies suggest that the anti-inflammatory effect of antioxidants found in nuts and green vegetables, such as spinach, broccoli and Brussels sprouts, which are also rich in vitamins C and E, may have a protective effect against Alzheimer's.

Arthritis

Again, diet seems to be very helpful in managing arthritis, especially osteo-arthritis (osteoarthritis is the form associated with wear and tear, while rheumatoid arthritis is a totally separate, autoimmune disease).

Simply being overweight already puts a strain on joints, especially the weight-bearing ones. Imagine what's happening when your knees, hips and ankles have to absorb an extra 22.5–27kg (50–60lb) of impact every time your foot hits the ground? Try lifting a 22.5kg (50lb) weight and you'll see what your poor body is coping with. Don't make your joints work any harder than they have to, and your joints will thank you for it. Not surprisingly, overweight and obese people account for the majority of hip and knee-replacement surgeries.

Also, some of the omega-3 essential fatty acids, found in oily fish and certain seeds and recommended by the Gi Diet, can help prevent and relieve osteoarthritis.

SUPPLEMENTS

A lot of people waste money on supplements. Most of us get at least the minimum recommended levels of most vitamins and minerals from our diet. There is increasing evidence, however, that the usual RDA (recommended daily allowance) may be insufficient in certain specific instances. This is a dynamic and fascinating area of nutrition research and very susceptible to change as new data pours in on a daily basis.

Based on our present knowledge, here are some guidelines that may be helpful.

Vitamin C

This is certainly the most popular vitamin on the market, mainly because of its reputation for preventing and curing colds. Although there is little evidence to support that particular claim, we do know that vitamin C is critical for the functioning of muscles, ligaments and joints.

While the Gi Diet, with its emphasis on fresh fruit and vegetables, will certainly cover your basic vitamin-C requirements, a top-up through a good quality one-a-day multivitamin may help.

B vitamins

There is growing evidence that vitamin B, or more specifically vitamins B6, B12 and folic acid, are key ingredients in combating a chemical called homocysteine, which attacks your arteries. This substance is triggered by the digestion of animal protein, which again suggests that high-protein diets can be dangerous to your health.

Because excessive doses of some B vitamins can be dangerous, the levels in most one-a-day multivitamins (20mcg B12, 2mg B6, 400mcg folic acid) are quite sufficient as a top-up to any possible deficiencies in your diet. You don't need to take B vitamins individually.

Vitamin D

Vitamin D is the true sunshine vitamin, and not vitamin C as adverts suggest. Although vitamin D is found in milk and fatty fish such as salmon, our body can also produce vitamin D itself when exposed to sunshine.

But for most of us, sunshine is a scarce commodity in winter, and, since we should be lathered in sunscreen during our all-too-brief summer, we are unable to capitalise on this vitamin self-generation.

Vitamin D is important because it facilitates the processing of calcium for the bones. This is critical for people over fifty, especially women, in order to prevent the bone-thinning disease osteoporosis. Equally important a shortage of vitamin D has recently been linked to several major cancers.

Again, the Gi Diet, with its emphasis on low-fat milk and fish, will help, but this is one instance where a vitamin D supplement of 1,000 IU is almost certainly a good idea.

Vitamin E

This became the wonder vitamin of the 1990s when it was suggested that it could reduce heart disease, Alzheimer's and certain cancers. There are many significant population studies currently under way, though recent heart-disease reports have been somewhat contradictory. Until there is more clarification on the role of this vitamin in our health, the Gi Diet will give you a sufficient supply of vitamin E, which is found in vegetable oils and nuts (both also sources of 'good' fat).

Fish oil

There is one oil in particular that has been found to have significant positive health benefits, particularly for your heart. The oil is called omega-3, and it is a fatty acid found primarily in oily fish, salmon in particular, but also mackerel, fresh tuna, sardines, pilchards and trout. You can also get omega-3 from rapeseed and flaxseed. If you are at risk of heart disease or stroke, then a daily fish oil capsule is a sensible option. The research evidence supporting omega-3 is overwhelming and much of it is Canadian, stemming from studies of the Inuit, who do not eat what we consider a heart-healthy diet, with loads of animal fat and virtually no fruit or vegetables. However, the seal and cold water fish they consume, rich in omega-3, appears to give them protection against heart disease.

Supplement summary
• The Gi Diet almost certainly contains sufficient vitamins to meet your daily needs. However, if you are at all concerned, a one-a-day multivitamin offers cheap and risk-free insurance.
• The role of vitamin C is uncertain, but keep your ears and eyes open to new research on this front.
• If heart health is a particular concern, omega-3-oil capsules are a good idea.
• An extra vitamin-D supplement is almost certainly worthwhile, particularly for women.

Appendix I
COMPLETE Gi DIET FOOD GUIDE

RED	YELLOW	GREEN
BEANS		**BEANS**
Broad		Black · Lima
		Black eyed · Mung
		Butter · Pigeon
		Chickpeas · Pinto
		Haricot/Navy · Romano
		Italian · Soy
		Kidney · Split
		Lentils
BEANS (TINNED)		**BEANS (TINNED)**
Baked beans with pork		Baked beans (low-fat)
Refried beans		Mixed salad beans
		Most varieties
		Vegetarian chilli

BEVERAGES

Alcoholic drinks
Coconut milk
Fruit drinks
Milk (whole)
Regular coffee
Regular soft drinks
Rice milk
Sweetened juice

BEVERAGES

Diet soft drinks (caffeinated)
Milk (semi-skimmed)
Red wine
Unsweetened fruit juices:
Apple
Cranberry
Grapefruit
Orange
Pear
Pineapple
Vegetable juice cocktails (e.g. V8)

BEVERAGES

Bottled water
Decaffeinated coffee
(with skimmed milk,
no sugar)
Diet soft drinks (no caffeine)
Herbal teas
Light instant chocolate
Milk (skimmed)
Soya milk (low-fat, plain)
Tea (with skimmed
milk, no sugar)

BREADS

100% stone-ground
wholemeal*
Homemade muffins
Wholegrain, high-fibre
breads (2½ to 3g of fibre per slice)*
Crispbreads (high-fibre) *

*Limit portions. See p.35

BREADS

Crispbread with fibre
Pitta (wholemeal)
Wholegrain breads

BREADS

Bagels
Baguettes/Croissants
Cereal/Granola bars
Crispbreads
Doughnuts
Hamburger buns
Hot dog buns
Kaiser rolls
Melba toast
Muffins
Pancakes/Waffles
Pizza
Stuffing
Tortillas
White bread

CEREALS

All cold cereals except those listed as yellow or green-light
Granola
Instant/quick cook porridge oats
Millet
Muesli (commercial)

CEREAL GRAINS

Almond flour
Amaranth
Couscous
Croutons
Millet
Polenta
Rice (short-grain, white, instant)
Rice cakes
Rice noodles

CEREALS

Shredded Wheat Bran

CEREAL GRAINS

Corn
Corn flour
Spelt
Wholemeal couscous

CEREALS

All-Bran
Alpen Crunchy Bran
High-Fibre Bran
Oat bran
Porridge oats (traditional large-flake e.g. Jordan's)
100% Bran
Soya protein powder
Steel-cut oats

CEREAL GRAINS

Arrowroot flour
Barley
Buckwheat bulgur
Bulgur
Gram flour
Kamut (not puffed)
Kasha (toasted buckwheat)
Quinoa
Rice (basmati, wild, brown, long-grain)
Soya protein powder
Wheat berries
Wheatgrain

CONDIMENTS/SEASONINGS

Croutons
Ketchup
Mayonnaise
Tartar sauce

DAIRY

Almond milk
Cheese
Chocolate milk
Cottage cheese (regular)
Cream
Cream cheese
Evaporated milk
Goats' milk
Milk (whole)
Rice milk
Sour cream
Yoghurt (regular)
Yoghurt (low fat)

CONDIMENTS/SEASONINGS

Mayonnaise (light)

DAIRY

Cheese (low fat)
Cream cheese (light)
Crème fraîche (low fat)
Ice cream (low fat)
Frozen yoghurt (low fat, low sugar)
Milk (semi-skimmed)
Soft margarine (non-hydrogenated)
Sour cream (light)
Sour cream (fat free)

CONDIMENTS/SEASONINGS

Chilli powder
Extracts (vanilla etc.)
Flavoured vinegars/sauces
Garlic
Herbs/Spices
Horseradish
Hummus
Lemon/lime juice
Mayonnaise (fat free)
Mustard
Peppers (all types)
Salsa (low sugar)
Soy sauce (low sodium)
Teriyaki sauce
Worcestershire sauce

DAIRY

Almond milk (low fat)
Buttermilk (skimmed low fat)
Cheese (fat free)
Cottage cheese (low fat or fat free)
Fruit yoghurt (fat free/with sweetener)
Ice cream (low fat and no added sugar, e.g. Wall's Soft Scoop Light)
Milk (skimmed)
Laughing Cow cheese (light)
Boursin cheese (light)
Soy cheese (low fat)
Soya milk (plain, low fat)
Soy/whey protein powder

FATS/OILS/DRESSINGS

Butter

Coconut oil

Hard margarine

Lard

Mayonnaise

Palm oil

Peanut butter (regular and light)

Salad dressings (regular)

Tropical oils

Vegetable shortening

*Limit portions. See p.35

FATS/OILS/DRESSINGS

Corn oil

Mayonnaise (light)

Most nuts

100% Peanut butter*

Peanut oil

Salad dressings (light)

Sesame oil

Soft margarine (non-hydrogenated)

Soy oil

Sunflower oil

Vegetable oils

FATS/OILS/DRESSINGS

Flaxseed oil*

Mayonnaise (low-fat/low sugar)

Olive oil*

Rapeseed oil*

Salad dressings (low fat/low sugar)

Soft margarine (non-hydrogenated, light)*

Vegetable oil sprays

Vinaigrette

FRUITS–FRESH

Cantaloupe melon
Dates
Honeydew melon
Kumquats
Watermelon

FRUITS–FRESH

Apricots (fresh)
Bananas
Figs
Kiwi
Mangoes
Papaya
Persimmon
Pineapple
Pomegranate

FRUITS–FRESH

Apples
Avocado (¼ per serving)
Blackberries
Blueberries
Cherries
Grapefruit
Grapes
Guavas
Lemons
Limes
Nectarines
Oranges
Peaches
Pears
Plums
Raspberries
Rhubarb
Strawberries

FRUITS – BOTTLED, TINNED, FROZEN, DRIED

All tinned fruit in syrup

Apple purée containing sugar

Most dried fruit*

*For baking, it is OK to use a modest amount of dried fruit

FRUIT SPREADS

Regular fruit spreads

FRUIT JUICES

Fruit drinks

Sweetened juices

Prune

Watermelon

FRUITS – BOTTLED, TINNED, FROZEN, DRIED

Dried apricots

Dried cranberries

Fruit cocktail in juice

Peaches/pears in syrup

Prunes

FRUIT SPREADS

FRUIT JUICES

Apple (unsweetened)

Cranberry (unsweetened)

Grapefruit (unsweetened)

Orange (unsweetened)

Pear (unsweetened)

Pineapple (unsweetened)

FRUITS – BOTTLED, TINNED, FROZEN, DRIED

Apple sauce (no sugar, e.g. Clearspring Organic)

Apple purée

Dried apples

Frozen berries

Mandarin oranges

Peaches in juice or water

FRUIT SPREADS

Extra fruit/low-sugar spreads

Fruit as first ingredient

FRUIT JUICES

Eat the fruit rather than drink the juice

MEAT, POULTRY, FISH, EGGS AND SOY

Boiled ham

Fish/shellfish (breaded/battered)

Hamburgers

Hot dogs

Minced beef (more than 10% fat)

Processed meats

Regular bacon

Sausages

Sushi (it's the rice)

Whole regular eggs

Pâté

Offal

MEAT, POULTRY, FISH, EGGS AND SOY

Chicken/turkey leg

Fish tinned in oil

Flank steak

Lamb (tenderloin, centre loin chop)

Minced beef (lean)

Pork (fore shank, leg shank, centre cut, loin chop)

Sirloin tip

Sirloin steak

Turkey bacon

Whole omega-3 eggs (e.g. Columbus)

MEAT, POULTRY, FISH, EGGS AND SOY

All seafood, fresh, frozen or tinned

Back bacon

Beef (top round steak, eye round steak)

Chicken breast (skinless)

Egg whites

Lean deli ham

Minced beef (extra lean)

Pork tenderloin

Quorn

Rabbit

Sashimi

Smoked salmon/trout

Soy/whey protein powder

Tofu

Turkey breast (skinless)

Veal (cutlet, rib roast, blade steak)

Venison

PASTA

All tinned pastas
Gnocchi
Macaroni and cheese
Noodles (tinned)
Pasta filled with cheese or meat

PASTA SAUCES

Alfredo
Sauces with added meat or cheese
Sauces with added sugar or sucrose

PASTA

Rice noodles

PASTA SAUCES

Sauces with vegetables

PASTA

Capellini
Cellophane noodles (mung bean)
Fettuccine
Linguine
Macaroni
Penne
Rigatoni
Spaghetti
Vermicelli

PASTA SAUCES

Light sauces with or without
vegetables (no added sugar)

SNACKS

Bagels
Biscuits
Bread
Chocolates and sweets
Coconuts
Cookies
Crisps/pretzels
Doughnuts
French fries
Ice cream
Jelly (all varieties)
Mixed dried fruit and nuts
Muffins (commercial)
Peanut butter (regular)
Popcorn (regular)
Raisins
Rice cakes
Sorbet
Tortilla chips

*Limit portions. See p.35

SNACKS

Bananas
Dark chocolate (70% cocoa)*
Ice cream (low fat)
Most nuts*
Peanut butter (100% peanuts)
Popcorn (light, microwaveable)

*Limit portions. See p.35

SNACKS

Almonds*
Apple purée (unsweetened)
Canned fruits
Cottage cheese (1% or fat free)
Food bars (12–15g protein; 4–5g fat e.g. Myoplex/Slim-Fast*)
Fruit yogurt (fat free/ with sweetener)
Hazelnuts*
Ice cream (low fat and no added sugar e.g. Wall's Soft Scoop Light)
Marmite**
Most fresh fruit
Most fresh vegetables
Most seeds
Nuts (see fats and oils)*
Soy nuts*
Tinned peaches/pears in juice or water
Vegemite**

*Limit portions. See p.35
**Caution: high sodium

SOUPS

All cream-based soups
Puréed vegetable
Tinned black bean
Tinned green pea
Tinned split pea

SUGAR AND SWEETENERS

Corn syrup
Glucose
Honey
Molasses
Sugar (all types)
Treacle

SOUPS

Tinned chicken noodle
Tinned lentil
Tinned tomato

SUGAR AND SWEETENERS

Fructose
Sugar alcohols

SOUPS

All homemade soups made with green-light ingredients

Chunky bean and vegetable soups (e.g. Baxter's Healthy Choice)

SUGAR AND SWEETENERS

Aspartame
Hermesetas Gold
Splenda®
Stevia®

TINNED/BOTTLED VEGETABLES

Roasted red peppers
Tinned/bottled vegetables
Tinned tomatoes
Tomato purée

VEGETABLES

Broad beans
French fries
Hash browns
Parsnips
Potatoes (instant)
Potatoes (mashed or baked)
Swede
Turnip

VEGETABLES

Artichokes
Beets
Corn
Potatoes (boiled)
Pumpkin
Squash
Sweet potatoes
Yams

VEGETABLES

Alfalfa sprouts
Asparagus
Aubergine
Beans (green/runner)
Bok choy
Broccoli
Brussels sprouts
Cabbage
Capers
Carrots
Cauliflower
Celery
Collard greens
Courgettes
Cucumber
Fennel
Kale
Leeks
Lettuce
Mangetout
Mushrooms
Mustard greens
Okra
Olives
Onions
Parsley
Peas
Peppers
Peppers (chillies)
Pickles
Potatoes (new/small)
Radicchio
Radishes
Sauerkraut
Spinach
Spring onions
Sugar snap peas
Swiss chard
Tomatoes

Appendix II

GI DIET SHOPPING LIST

FRIDGE/FREEZER

Dairy
Milk (skimmed)
Yoghurt (with sweetener)
Buttermilk
Cottage cheese (low-fat)
Frozen yoghurt (fat-free with no added sugar)
Sorbet (sugar-free)

Meat/poultry/fish/eggs
Ham/turkey/chicken (lean deli)
Pork loin
Extra-lean minced beef
Chicken breast (skinless)
Turkey breast (skinless)
Veal
Omega-3 eggs
All fish and seafood (no batter or breading)

Fats/spreads
Margarine (light)
Mayonnaise (low/no-fat)

Fruit
Apples
Blueberries
Blackberries
Cherries
Grapes
Grapefruit

Vegetables
Asparagus
Aubergine
Beans (green/French)
Broccoli
Cabbage
Carrots
Cauliflower
Celery
Courgettes
Cucumber
Leeks
Lettuce
Mange tout
Mushrooms
Olives
Onions
Peppers
Potatoes (new, small only)
Spinach
Tomatoes

PANTRY

Baking/cooking
Wholemeal flour
Baking powder/soda
Cocoa
Wheat/oat bran
Sliced almonds
Dried apricots

Bread
100% whole wheat

Cereals
Porridge (large-flake)
All-Bran
High-Fibre Bran

Beans (canned)
Most varieties
Baked beans (low-fat)
Mixed salad beans
Vegetarian chilli

Fruit (canned)
Apple purée (no sugar)
Peaches in juice or water
Pears in juice or water
Mandarin oranges in juice (not syrup)

Rice
Basmati

Pasta
Capellini
Fettuccine
Macaroni
Penne
Spaghetti
Vermicelli

Pasta Sauces (vegetable-based only)
Dolmio Original Light

Oils
Olive oil
Rapeseed oil
Vegetable-oil spray

Salad dressings
Vinaigrette

Seasonings
Spices/herbs
Flavoured vinegars/sauces

Soups
Baxter's Healthy Choice

Sweeteners
Splenda®
Hermesetas (and other artificial sweeteners)

Food bars
Myoplex
Slim-Fast

Nuts
Almonds

Drinks
Diet soft drinks
Soda water
Coffee/tea
Bottled water

Appendix III

GI DIET DINING OUT TIPS

BREAKFAST – GREEN-LIGHT

All-Bran
Egg whites – omelette
Egg whites – scrambled
Fruit
Porridge oats
Yoghurt (low-fat)

BREAKFAST – RED-LIGHT

Cold cereals
Bacon/sausage
Eggs
Scones
Pancakes/waffles

LUNCH – GREEN-LIGHT

Meats – deli-style ham/chicken/
turkey breast
Pasta – ¼ plate maximum
Salads – low-fat (dressing on the side)
Sandwiches – open-faced
whole wheat
Soups – chunky vegetable/bean
Vegetables
Wraps – ½ wholemeal pita, no mayon-
naise

LUNCH – RED-LIGHT

Bakery products
Butter/mayonnaise
Cheese
Fast food
Pasta-based meals
Pizza/bread/bagels
Potatoes (replace with double
vegetables)

DINNER – GREEN-LIGHT

Chicken/turkey (no skin)
Fruit
Pasta – ¼ plate
Rice (basmati, brown, wild, long-grain)
– ¼ plate
Salads – low-fat (dressing on the side)
Seafood – not breaded or battered
Soups – chunky vegetable/bean
Vegetables

DINNER – RED-LIGHT

Beef/lamb/pork
Bread
Butter/mayonnaise
Caesar salad
Potatoes (replace with double
vegetables)
Puddings
Soups – cream based

SNACKS – GREEN-LIGHT

Almonds
Food bar – ½ of one
Fresh fruit
Hazelnuts
Yoghurt – 'diet'

SNACKS – RED-LIGHT

Crisps, all types
Biscuits/cakes/scones
Popcorn, regular

Appendix IV

EXERCISE CALORIE COUNTER

(Figures indicate calories burned in 30 minutes.)

YOUR WEIGHT (IN LB):	130	160	200
GYM AND HOME ACTIVITIES			
Aerobics: low impact	172	211	264
Aerobics: high impact	218	269	336
Aerobics, step: low impact	218	269	336
Aerobics, step: high impact	312	384	480
Aerobics: water	125	154	192
Bicycling, stationary: moderate	218	269	336
Bicycling, stationary: vigorous	328	403	504
Circuit training: general	250	307	384
Rowing, stationary: moderate	218	269	336
Rowing, stationary: vigorous	265	326	408
Ski machine: general	296	365	456
Stair step machine: general	187	230	288
Weightlifting: general	94	115	144
Weightlifting: vigorous	187	230	288
TRAINING ACTIVITIES			
Basketball: playing a game	250	307	384
Basketball: wheelchair	203	250	312
Bicycling: BMX or mountain	265	326	408
Bicycling: 12–13.9 mph	250	307	384
Bicycling: 14–15.9 mph	312	384	480
Boxing: sparring	281	346	432
Football: competitive	281	346	432
Football: general	250	307	384
Frisbee	94	115	144
Golf: carrying clubs	172	211	264
Golf: using cart	109	134	168
Gymnastics: general	125	154	192
Handball: general	374	461	576
Hiking: cross-country	187	230	288
Horse riding: general	125	154	192
Ice skating: general	218	269	336
Martial arts: general	312	384	480
Racquetball: competitive	312	384	480

Activity			
Racquetball: casual, general	218	269	336
Rock climbing: ascending	343	422	528
Rock climbing: repelling	250	307	384
Rollerblading	218	269	336
Running: 5 mph (12 min/mile)	250	307	384
Running: 5.2 mph (11.5 min/mile)	281	346	432
Running: 6 mph (10 min/mile)	312	384	480
Running: 6.7 mph (9 min/mile)	343	422	528
Running: 7.5 mph (8 min/mile)	390	480	600
Running: 8.6 mph (7 min/mile)	452	557	696
Running: 10 mph (6 min/mile)	515	634	792
Running: pushing wheelchair, marathon wheeling	250	307	384
Running: cross-country	281	346	432
Skiing: cross-country	250	307	384
Skiing: downhill	187	230	288
Skipping	312	384	480
Snowshoeing	250	307	384
Softball: general play	156	192	240
Swimming: general	187	230	288
Tennis: general	218	269	336
Volleyball: non-competitive, general play	94	115	144
Volleyball: competitive, gymnasium play	125	154	192
Volleyball: beach	250	307	384
Walk: 3.5 mph (17 min/mile)	125	154	192
Walk: 4 mph (15 min/mile)	140	173	216
Walk: 4.5 mph (13 min/mile)	156	192	240
Walk/jog: jog more than 10 min.	187	230	288
Water Polo	312	384	480
Waterskiing	187	230	288
Whitewater: rafting, kayaking	156	192	240

DAILY LIFE ACTIVITIES

Activity			
Children's games: hopscotch etc.	156	192	240
Chopping and splitting wood	187	230	288
Gardening: general	140	173	216
House cleaning: general	109	134	168
Mowing lawn: push, hand	172	211	264
Mowing lawn: push, power	140	173	216
Raking lawn	125	154	192
Sex: moderate effort		47	58	72
Shovelling snow: by hand	187	230	288

Appendix V

THE TEN GOLDEN GI DIET RULES

1. Eat three meals and three snacks every day. Don't skip meals – breakfast is particularly important.

2. Stick with green-light products only in Phase I.

3. Always ensure that each meal contains the appropriate measure of carbohydrates, protein and fat.

4. Eat at least three times more vegetables and fruit than usual.

5. When it comes to food, quantity is as important as quality. Especially if you're in Phase I, you'll probably need to shrink your usual portions, particularly of meat, pasta and rice.

6. Drink plenty of fluids, preferably water.

7. Introduce more activity into your everyday life; for example, get off the bus two stops early and use the stairs rather than the lift or escalator.

8. Find a friend to join you for mutual support.

9. Set realistic goals and record your progress to reinforce your sense of achievement.

10. Don't view this as a diet. It's the basis of how you will eat for the rest of your life.

Appendix VI

GI DIET WEEKLY WEIGHT AND WAIST LOG

WEEK	DATE	WEIGHT	WAIST	COMMENTS
1				
2				
3				
4				
5				
6				
7				
8				
9				
10				
11				
12				
13				
14				
15				
16				
17				
18				
19				
20				

Appendix VII

GI DIET EXERCISE LOG

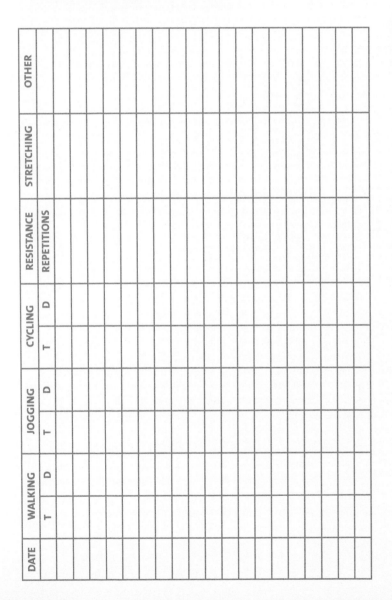

DATE	WALKING		JOGGING		CYCLING		RESISTANCE	STRETCHING	OTHER
	T	D	T	D	T	D	REPETITIONS		

Readers' Stories

'From a weight of 24 stone 4 pounds I now weigh exactly 14 stone. That is a total loss in one full year of 10 stone 4 pounds! I am delighted with how the Gi Diet has changed my life. I had a full medical with the doctor a month ago. My cholesterol levels are fine and blood pressure has gone from on the high side to perfect levels. My doctor is amazed and regards my health as a complete turnaround. My life is completely different as my confidence and self esteem have returned.' **Martin**.

'I weighed 14 stone. My doctor told me I needed to go on high blood pressure medicine, but I convinced her to let me try to lower my blood pressure naturally. She gave me two months. Two weeks later I read an article in Woman's World about your diet, and in three days I lost three pounds! I knew I had to buy the book. It is now one year later and I weigh 9 stone 11 pounds, my blood pressure is perfect without medicine and I have lost approximately 40 inches. As an added bonus, people see how good I look and feel and they try it too. I feel so much better; I will never go back to my old bad eating habits.' **Jeri**.

'I gained 5 stone 10 pounds when I was pregnant with my first child. Not used to being overweight, I needed to get the weight off but also learn about nutrition, since I was planning to nurse my baby as well. My sister, a personal trainer, came across your book, bought it and said that it was simple, made sense, and was something easy enough for me to follow. The education and resources that you provided me have been invaluable, I am back in my business suits (what a cost saving, not having to by new ones) and am 5 pounds less than when I got pregnant. I now feel the need to educate my friends, recommend your book and will raise a son with good eating habits. I am looking forward to gaining only minimal weight the next pregnancy. Thank you very much for making such a positive change in my life.' **Beth**

I started the Gi Diet after my doctor informed me that I had four major problems with my health. My blood pressure, cholesterol and weight (over 20 stone) were dangerously high, in addition to which I had type 2 diabetes. Well, 9 months have past since I started the Gi Diet and I now weigh under 14 stone and all the above mentioned health problems are under control or no longer exist. I have lost over 6 stone and my doctor now calls me his star patient.' **Gail**.

Index

alcohol 44, 49, 53, 115, 128
Alzheimer's disease 7, 129, 134
antioxidants 38, 48, 134
apples 108, 109
arthritis 129, 135, 136

bacon 37, 38, 40, 52, 56, 76, 109
beans (legumes) 8, 9, 43, 108, 138, 151
beef:
  beef chilli 72
  beef cutlets in mushroom gravy 76, 81
  mushroom, barley and beef soup 76, 83
berry crumble 76, 81–2
biscotti, savoury 73–4, 76
black bean soup, smoky 78, 101
blood sugar 14, 15, 114
BMI:
  finding your 20–1
  setting your target 24–5, 114
  table 22–3
bread 9, 75, 76, 108, 140, 151
breakfast 59–61, 76, 77, 78, 116, 127
brownies, pecan 78, 107, 114

calories 4, 10, 14, 28, 29, 33, 34, 35, 36, 37, 39, 45, 47, 48, 49, 51, 53, 55, 56, 108, 109, 110, 115, 127
  calculating 4, 25
  exercise and 117, 118, 120, 122, 123, 124, 125, 126, 153–4
  fat and 6, 7
  food labels and 28, 30
  traffic-light system and 16
cancer 7, 134
carbohydrates 11–12, 34, 43–4, 47
cereals 34, 35, 53, 59–60, 109, 141, 151
charting your progress 26
cheese 7, 31
  cheese blintzes 62
  cottage cheese 52, 65, 109
  escarole and berry salad with herb and lemon vinaigrette and blue cheese 65
  tomato and cheese fish 67–8
  yoghurt cheese 86, 112
chicken:
  barbecue chicken 76, 84
  chicken curry 70
  chicken tagine 78, 106
  Italian chicken 70
  open-faced chicken reuben sandwich 78, 100
  white chicken chilli 76, 89–90
Chinese food 16, 54
chocolate 73, 77, 78, 113, 114, 128
  chocolate drop cookies 78, 98, 114
cholesterol 8, 29, 36, 37, 110, 131, 132
coffee and tea 9, 34, 38, 48, 54, 76, 77, 78
coleslaw, tangy red-and-green 87–8
cookies:
  apple-sauce cookies 77, 78, 90
  chocolate drop cookies 78, 98, 114
cooking 57–8
cottage cheese and fruit 52, 65, 109
courgette coins, oven-baked 69
crab salad in tomato shells 76, 80
cravings, food 17, 113–14

dairy 8, 32, 37, 142, 151
desserts 40, 45, 52, 54
diabetes 130, 133
diets 8, 24–5
dining out tips 152 see also restaurants
dinner 42–50
  Phase I 76, 77, 78
  Phase II 128
  recipes 66–72
dressings 33, 143, 151
drinks/beverages 34, 48–9, 110, 139, 151 see also alcohol

eggs 37, 109, 146
energy bars 47, 109
energy increase 18–19
exercise 117–25, 153–4, 157

fast food 55–6
fat, losing 18–23 see also weight loss
fats 6–7, 8, 9, 28–9, 33, 143, 151
fibre 29
fish 8, 71, 134, 146
  oil 8, 31, 136–7
  quick fish steaks with tomato-chickpea relish 78, 102
  supermarket counter 32
  tomato and cheese fish 67–8
food bars 109, 151
frozen food 31, 43, 44
fruit 10, 37, 76, 144, 145
  cottage cheese and fruit 52, 65
  grilled fruit kebabs with a lemon-yoghurt sauce 78, 103
  morning glory poached fruit 77, 94
frying pans, non-stick 57–8

Gi Diet:
  complete food guide 138–50
  exercise log 157
  losing weight on the 18–23
  Phase I - the 7-day plan 76–8, 79–108
  Phase II 126–8
  ten golden rules of 155
  weekly weight and waist log 156
Glycemic Index (GI) 13–17
grapefruit 109
green-light foods 16, 29
  at breakfast 36
  cooking 57
  fast food 55
  food guide 138–50
  glossary of 108–12
  on holiday 116
  labels and 30
  meal planning 60
  at parties 115–16
  portions 34, 35
  servings, recommended 35
  shopping for 26, 27, 31, 32, 33, 34, 35, 36, 37, 38, 39, 40, 42, 44, 45, 46, 47, 49, 69
grill pan/indoor grill 58

ham and lentil soup 77, 95
hamburgers 109
health 6, 7, 8, 9, 16, 19 exercise and see exercise
  GI Diet and 129–31
heart disease and stroke 130–1
holidays 116
hummus, roasted red pepper 78, 105, 115-16
hyperglycaemia 15
hypertension 131–2

ice cream 114
Indian and South Asian food 55
insulin 15, 32

juices 37, 48, 49, 110, 127 see also drinks/beverages

labels, what to look for on 28–30
lemon squares, creamy 74
lunch 9, 39–41, 51–2, 61–5, 76, 77, 78, 127

meal planning 58
meat 109, 146
  at restaurants 54
  recipes 71
  red 42
  shopping list 151
  supermarket counter 31
milk 110
  skimmed 49, 109
  soya 49
motivation 113–16
muesli, breakfast 76, 82
mushroom, barley and beef
  soup 76, 83

nuts and seeds 10, 33, 110,
  116, 151

oat bran 110
oatmeal, homey 78, 104
obesity 4, 6, 7, 129, 130, 133
oils 7, 8, 33, 53, 143, 151
olive oil 8, 33
omega-3 8, 31, 134, 137
omelette 60–1
oranges 110

pancakes, buttermilk 77, 87
parties and celebrations
  115–16
pasta 9, 11, 16, 32, 34, 44, 52,
  55, 110, 147
paté, smoked trout 77, 89
peach meringue 77, 93
peaches 110
pears 100
  almond crusted 97
  poached 85–6
pecan brownies 78, 107, 114
peppers, stuffed 66
Phase I 16, 24, 26, 27, 38, 45,
  76–8, 79–108, 114
Phase II 16, 24, 26, 126–8
porridge 76, 79, 110
portions, perfect 34–5
potatoes 16, 34, 44, 54, 110–11
poultry 42–3, 54, 69, 146
prawns, chilli-lime tiger 63
protein 8–9, 29
  animal 8, 9, 43
  at dinner 42
  lean 14
  sources of 8, 9–10
  vegetable 9, 10, 43

Quorn 31

recipes:
  breakfast 59–61
  lunch 62–5
  dinner 66–75
  7 day plan 79–108
red-light foods:
  blood sugar and 114
  bread 108

breakfast 36, 37
chocolate 128
clearing out 27
cooking 57
  at dinner 44
  fast-food 55
  holidays and 116
  at lunch 51
  at parties 115
  rice 111
  shopping and 16, 27, 30, 31,
    32, 33, 34
  snacks 17, 47
restaurants 16, 53–4, 116, 152
rice 16, 33, 34, 44, 54, 55, 111, 151

salad 9, 33, 39, 111
  barbecue-chicken salad
    76, 84
  crab salad in tomato shells
    76, 80
  escarole and berry salad
    with herb and lemon vinai-
    grette and blue cheese 65
  lunchtime salad 52
  salad and vinaigrette,
    everyday 63
salmon, grilled pesto with
  asparagus 76, 85
sandwich bars 52–3
sandwiches 51–2, 61
  open-faced chicken reuben
    sandwich 78, 100
  open-faced lunch sandwich
    77, 78, 88
seafood 9, 34, 42, 57, 80
seasonings 151
serving sizes 28, 31, 32, 42,
  44, 108, 109, 126, 127 see also
  portions
shepherd's pie, vegetarian
  92–3
shopping 27–34, 151
slow-release fuels, finding
  the 13–15
smoking 130
snacks 33, 47–8, 73–5, 148
  Phase I 76, 77, 78
  Phase II 128
sodium (salt) 29–30
soft drinks 34, 49, 114, 115
soups 39, 53, 61, 76, 149
  chilled spinach and water-
    cress soup 99–100
  ham and lentil soup 77, 95
  haricot bean soup 79
  minestrone soup 77, 91–2
  mushroom barley and beef
    soup 76, 83
  smoky black bean soup 78,
    101
  Tuscan white bean soup
    78, 104
soy sauce 116, 146
soya 9, 10, 31, 34, 43, 49, 110

soya milk 49, 110
spreads 36
steak 7, 42, 71, 132
sugar 12, 13, 27, 29, 31, 32, 33, 34,
  35, 36, 37, 38, 45, 47, 48, 49,
  52, 54, 55, 56, 108, 109, 111,
  128, 133, 149 see also blood
  sugar
supermarkets 30–4
supplements 135–7 see also
  vitamins
sweeteners 33–4, 48, 111,
  149, 151

ten golden rules 155
textured vegetable protein
  (TVP) 31, 43
Thai food 16, 77
Thai-style tofu and broccoli
  77, 96
toast 9, 35, 76, 77, 91
tofu 8, 10, 31, 34, 43, 77, 96
tomatoes 32, 52, 68
traffic-light system 4, 16–17
  breakfast 38–9
  dinner 45–6
  drinks 49
  food guide 138–50
  lunch 40–1
  see also green-light, red-
  light and yellow-light foods
  trout paté, smoked 89

vegetables 10, 17, 29, 30, 31, 32,
  34, 35, 53, 115, 134, 150
  at dinner 42, 44
  shopping list 151
  supermarket aisle 30
vegetarians 31, 34, 43, 57, 60,
  72, 77, 92–3
vinaigrette 33, 52, 63, 64
vitamins 17, 30, 31, 42, 134, 135,
  136, 137

waist measurement 21–2, 26,
  37, 56, 110, 156
water 29, 48, 49, 50, 53, 115 see
  also drinks/
  beverages
weight:
  how much should I weigh?
    19–20
  losing 18–23
  obesity 4, 6, 7, 129, 130, 133
  waist measurement 21–2,
    24, 26, 37, 56, 110, 156
  weekly weight and waist
    log 21–2, 26, 156
wheat 11, 29, 36, 38, 44, 53, 59,
  71, 77, 99, 108

yellow-light foods 16, 17, 26, 27,
  33, 71, 109, 126, 127
yoghurt 53, 77, 86, 111–12,
  114, 116